Cancer
and
Fishnet Stockings

Cancer
and
Fishnet Stockings

How Humor Helped Me Survive a Life-threatening Disease, the Loss of My Favorite Nail Polish...and Other Calamities

MARYANN GRAU

Foreword by Dr. Brian DiCarlo

ISBN: 978-1-7335909-0-7

A portion of the proceeds from this book will
be donated to the Pancreatic Cancer Action Network

Book Design by *the*BookDesigners

For Darlene, Joseph, Taylor and Chase

In the depth of winter
I finally learned
That within me there lay
An invincible summer

—Albert Camus

FOREWORD

When people ask me what I do for a living, and they hear I am an oncologist, they frequently respond with, "That must be a sad, depressing job." I often find it just the opposite. While it can bring sad situations, especially with diseases such as pancreatic cancer, I find it remarkable how rewarding and life-affirming my work can be. A day does not go by that I am not inspired by one of my patients, whether it be by motivation or reiteration of the preciousness of time in our lives.

When I first met Maryann Grau, I anticipated having one of the more difficult discussions in oncology—that of a diagnosis of pancreatic cancer. This is a dreaded diagnosis, and it is a disease that generally lives up to its terrible reputation. What I encountered, however, was a woman who viewed her new diagnosis with a remarkable level of clarity and understanding. Over the next couple of years, she taught me how to approach a potentially devastating disease with great courage, grace, and humor.

"Humor" may surprise you. It comes as a surprise to many, how much laughter I share with my patients, and how often they show me the importance of maintaining a healthy sense of humor. Those who do, tend to travel through their cancer journeys with less turbulence and anxiety. Maryann often made humorous remarks, but I didn't realize, during my fifteen to thirty- minute office visits with her, how genuinely funny she is—until I read her book.

Cancer and Fishnet Stockings will make you laugh and cry—sometimes from laughing. While Maryann's story details the often complicated and stressful medical system and the fear caused by a cancer diagnosis, it's full of the genuine humor she found in even this most difficult life circumstance.

This book inspires, motivates, engenders thought, and yes, makes you laugh. Above all, it will help others facing their own difficult cancer journeys. I intend to recommend it to all my patients.

—Dr. Brian DiCarlo, Oncologist

PREFACE

Cancer is no laughing matter. But this book isn't about cancer. It's about choices. When I was diagnosed with pancreatic cancer and made aware that my days were very likely numbered, the first thought that entered my mind was, *Maybe they're wrong.* Not about the low survivability rate for that kind of cancer—I knew it was a tough one to beat—but wrong about me. I didn't doubt the tumor's sincerity in its aim to do me in, but I wasn't going down without a fight!

Oh, I know I didn't look tough lying there weak, pale, and dripping with vomit, under a white sheet in the recovery room after the test that discovered the tumor. But sad as the news was, this was not my first battle in life, and I honestly didn't think it would be my last. I knew I could rely on some inner strength to help me make the right choices: courage over fear, hope over despair, and, more importantly, laughter over tears, because without the ability to laugh, the urge to surrender would be too strong.

The email updates I sent to family and friends throughout my treatment were penned straight from the heart and became the driving force behind this book. Recipients called those emails "inspiring," "entertaining," and, often, "hilarious." I called them "lifesavers," because every day I could write was a day I had outwitted that Angel of Death lurking just outside my door.

As I write this, the dishes are piling up in the sink, the plants are screaming for water, my phone needs charging, ditto my car battery (AAA is on the way) but I've a story to tell, so here I sit, staring at a blank page, and to hell with everything else.

So, you see? This book is not about cancer. It's about life. It's about love. It's about laughter. It's about me.

And maybe, it's about you.

ACKNOWLEDGMENTS

As much as I would like to take full credit for this book, I must confess that I had a great deal of help. So, it's only proper that I blame, I mean thank, those who talked me into giving up what had been a peaceful existence— leisurely walks along the coast, wine-tasting excursions, catching up on my reading, visiting family—and instead, chain, uh, devote myself to this arduous task for the last eighteen months. Now that it's done, I just want to do something normal again, like go outside!

Darlene Halaby and Taylor O'Sullivan offered tremendous encouragement every step of the way. When I was anxious for their feedback on my final draft, they read a digital version of the manuscript on an overnight business flight to Kenya. (Who does that?) And, the fact that they are my daughter and granddaughter had absolutely nothing to do with their eagerness to do so, I'm sure. (Love you, girls)

Mike Griffin, Christine Quinn, and Craig Wasson. These brave souls were the first to read through and edit my first draft. Each made corrections, provided guidance, gave positive comments that boosted my confidence, and led this starry-eyed author wanna-be to believe she actually had a book in the making.

Lisa Tanzman and I were enjoying lunch at Harmony Café (great pizza!) when I broke the news to her, and she immediately searched her brain for contacts in the publishing industry she thought might be helpful. Several chapters were then rushed off to New York and were quickly returned with advice that proved extremely valuable—self publish!

When I told Norb I was planning to write a book, his response was, "Of course you are!" If I had mentioned that I was planning to climb Mt. Kilimanjaro, I don't doubt I'd have heard the same response. When someone believes in you, he believes in you.

My dear friend, Jeannie Price, never tired of my reaching out to her almost daily for feedback, and I'm as confident as I could be, that this is *not* what drove her to move out of the state. I could always count on her blunt, but honest criticism, and I plan to send her a copy of the book—as soon as she gives me her new address in Arizona.

Di and Bill Civiello were early sounding boards,

too. They never hesitated to offer advice and suggestions, no matter how often I crossed the street and knocked on their door with the latest chapter in hand. Now that I think of it, they have since moved to Idaho. (Am I sensing a trend here?)

I want to thank everyone in my aerobics and strength training classes. Many of them were the first to suggest that I write the book and cheered me on throughout the entire process. I would think lovingly of them on those many long nights when I lay awake struggling over how to end a chapter or what title I should pick or...yes, lovingly.

I am grateful to the members of my writing group, the Rough Writers, for their patience in assisting a relative newcomer through the writing and publishing processes. Yikes! Did I make a lot of mistakes! But I'm thankful that I heard no finger-tapping around the table as I struggled through the reading of those first rough drafts. Their wisdom and kindness knew no bounds

I especially thank my oncologist, Dr. Brian DiCarlo, for championing the project from the start, for his glowing endorsement in the Foreword and, oh yes, for saving my life! I was relieved to know that the book had not caused him to reflect on the wisdom of doing so.

And my sincere thanks to you, dear reader, for shining your light, momentarily, on me.

CONTENTS

PART I: CANCER

Chapter 1: Harold's Pancakes 3

Chapter 2: Can This Be Happening to Me? 7

Chapter 3: You Can't Shop if You're Dead 15

Chapter 4: A Virgo With a Plan, Or Is That Redundant? 19

Chapter 5: Fishnet Stockings 25

Chapter 6: *Doctor Doom*: The Musical 29

Chapter 7: Ode to "The Californians" 33

Chapter 8: Meatballs and Helicopter Moms 37

Chapter 9: The Oncology Center 41

Chapter 10: Little Green What? 47

Chapter 11: Ali's Artichoke Ravioli…and More 51

Chapter 12: Chemo Buddy 55

Chapter 13: Grandchildren: Life's Greatest Reward 59

Chapter 14: Stripes or Checks? 65

Chapter 15: How Can I Help? 69

Chapter 16: Hair Today, Gone Tomorrow 73

Chapter 17: Legal Issues.. 77

Chapter 18: Bam! Zap! Kapow!... 81

Chapter 19: Spend All Your Kisses 85

Chapter 20: The Bald Spots 93

Chapter 21: False Alarm!.. 97

Chapter 22: Joy Is Not the Absence of Pain.............................. 101

Chapter 23: Frankenstein and Wine.. 105

Chapter 24: A Year of Living Dangerously 109

Chapter 25: Two to Five 113

Chapter 26: Dragon Slayer... 115

PART II: OTHER CALAMITIES

Chapter 27: Me and Galileo... 125

Chapter 28: Slaying the Dragon Slayer 129

Chapter 29: Bionic Woman.. 131

Chapter 30: I'm Alive, So Why Not Shop? 135

Chapter 31: It's My Body and I'll Cry If I Want To... 137

Chapter 32: Ducking Bullets... 141

Chapter 33: Fear Is a Reaction, Courage Is a Decision 145

Chapter 34: Speaking of Heaven 149

Chapter 35: Bucket List?.. 153

Chapter 36: A Dream 157

Chapter 37: I've Been Through Hell and I'm Not
Gonna Take It Anymore!... 161

Chapter 38: Should I Kill Myself or Have a Cup of Coffee?..... 165

Chapter 39: Spoiler Alert: I'm still Here 167

Chapter 40: R-E-S-P-E-C-T.. 169

Chapter 41: Never Give In, Never Give In,
Never, Never, Never! 173

Chapter 42: "Cancer Is Cool...," Said No One,
Anywhere, Ever!..177

Chapter 43: Harold's Pancake Recipe 181

1

Cancer

CHAPTER ONE

Harold's Pancakes

I must confess that facing the possibility of my own imminent death has me conjuring up the craziest thoughts. Why am I thinking about Harold? And his pancakes?

I don't know Harold. Never met him. But I've been making his pancakes since the early 70's when my friend Ralph shared that scrumptious recipe with me. They're made from scratch with buttermilk and sour cream, and they're the lightest pancakes on earth. When my kids were growing up, those fluffy treasures were a weekly treat; every Sunday morning...Harold's Pancakes! I take comfort in that thought now because I know my daughter and granddaughter will continue to make those pancakes long after I'm gone.

And maybe that's one of the ways a soul lives on after death.

For me, that could be soon, considering the news that was dumped on me this morning. Yes, I'm having pangs of sadness. And yes, I hope there is a place from which I might be able to look down and watch my girls smother those hot-off-the-griddle cakes in melted butter and warm Vermont maple syrup on Sunday mornings. Wouldn't that be sweet?

My good friend JoAnn loved the pancakes, too, and in 1985 when she decided to open a restaurant in Santa Barbara across from Stearns Wharf, she asked if she could put *my* pancakes on the menu. I was pretty sure Ralph, and probably Harold, too, had been dead for many years, and I didn't think recipes fell under any copyright protection, so I blurted out "absolutely," and they became "Maryann's Pancakes" to an unsuspecting clientele on the coast of California.

It occurs to me now that if there is a hereafter, I may soon have to atone for this brief lapse in moral character. But maybe it's not too late to set the record straight. I've always wanted to compile a cookbook of my favorite recipes, and if there's still enough time to complete that endeavor, I will include the pancake recipe and give Harold the full credit he deserves. Although—the thought crosses my mind—Harold probably pinched the recipe from someone else. And that's *his* problem to put right...if he hasn't already done so.

What about other possible misdeeds? Perhaps I can make amends for them, too. But I have the feeling I had better be darn quick about it.

CHAPTER 2

Can This Be Happening to Me?

I checked into Sierra Vista Medical center in San Luis Obispo at 6:00 a.m. as an outpatient, expecting I'd be out in time for lunch or an early dinner. Di—the dear friend who drove me into town—and I talked about stopping for lunch at Ruddell's Smokehouse in Cayucos on the way home. A small dive of a place only steps from the beach, it had been judged by *Sunset* magazine as one of the best eateries for fish on either coast, and we went regularly.

I've had some stomach issues lately (nothing to do with Ruddell's smoked chicken tacos, I'm sure), and Dr. Meiselman, my gastroenterologist, has planned a fairly invasive test to determine the source of pain just under my left breast. A previous test, an EGD (Esophagogastroduodenoscopy) examining the lining of the stomach and duodenum, revealed nothing, and I half expect this test—an ERCP (Endoscopic Retrograde Cholangiopancreatography)—to be a dud, too.

An ERCP is used to examine the gallbladder, liver, and pancreas. It involves a scope the size of a finger, a light, a contrast dye, and a camera with X-ray to check for the presence of disease. It is not commonly performed in the small, central California coastal community where I reside, but Dr. Meiselman hails from Chicago, where it is widely practiced. He's assured me he has done it many times. I'm not worried.

Di is in the waiting room, and I am behind a curtain in the pre-op area. A lovely young nurse helps me into a gown, leads me to a scale (*must I?*), and takes my temperature. After starting an IV, she offers me a warm blanket, which I readily accept. So far, so good. I check the wall clock. *Will we make it to lunch?*

"Someone will let us know when the doctor is ready, and you'll be taken down to the operating room," the nurse briefs me before drawing the curtain closed and moving on to the next patient.

I fill the time wondering just what the doctor has to do to get ready. *Finish his caramel latte? A quick refresher on how to perform this procedure? Last-minute check to see how the market is doing? Jeez, I hope it's up; I know how riled I get when the Dow takes a dive!* The curtain is yanked open, and a young, strapping orderly reaches for the foot of the gurney.

"Mrs. Grau, if you're all set, I'll take you down to

surgery now," he says in a far cheerier voice than the situation calls for.

"No thanks, I'm good," I respond, while drawing the blanket up over my head. He chuckles politely and begins to roll the gurney, wheels clacking, through hallways, past the cafeteria (*I smell bacon*), into an elevator, where he presses "down." In the basement, he rolls me over to a holding area just outside the operating room. "The doctor will be with you shortly," he says as he ambles away.

Why am I going into an operating room if this is only a "procedure?" I wonder. I'm still in a holding position when the anesthesiologist arrives. We barely exchange greetings before I advise him that I will need a heavy dose of anti-nausea medication because anesthesia always makes me vomit violently. *Oops! Did I actually just give advice to a doctor? Yup! His pursed lips are a dead giveaway.* "Anesthesia is administered based on the patient's weight, age, and the type of procedure," he says. And he assures me that "you will be just fine." I bite my lip rather than tell him I have heard that before.

As the pre-op drugs kick in, background noises begin to fade, and I drift happily to sleep. This is the part of anesthesia that I *do* enjoy! What seems like only minutes later, I awake in recovery, where, to everyone's dismay, it's obvious that the anti-nausea meds were not effective. Dr. Meiselman and Di, who had been called in from the waiting room, are standing over me on the right. A nurse on my left holds a bag under my chin, and another is wiping my face with a damp cloth. The doctor looks grim, and I begin to worry. *Maybe the mess I'm making of this room has him upset?*

"Maryann, we found a tumor in the pancreas," he tells me in a solemn voice.

My gut is still wrenching. I try to stem the bitter flow, take a quick breath, and ask hesitatingly, "Is it... *malignant?*"

I can tell by the way his face softens what the answer is. "We did several biopsies, and yes, unfortunately, they do prove positive for cancer."

I can feel the blood rush from my brain, but I do not pass out, surprisingly, as I have a history of fainting spells. Instead, an unexpected calm comes over me. Acceptance? Too soon. Denial? Not my nature.

But I know just enough about pancreatic cancer to know it is one of the hardest to cure and that the return rate is high. The vomiting continues.

Dr. Meiselman excuses himself and steps to a phone just outside the recovery room. Di and I exchange looks. She is a retired nurse and well-practiced at controlling her emotions in the presence of patients, but the hint of sadness in her eyes is unmistakable.

"Don't let them send me home like this," I plead with her.

"I won't," she assures me. I can hear Dr. Meiselman on the phone with my GP, Dr. Negri, recommending that he admit me to the hospital. I breathe a sigh of relief.

When the nausea subsides, I am wheeled into an unoccupied patient room. Seeing me settled, Di leaves, but not before discussing what I might need her to handle for me at home.

Then I am alone.

And I am suddenly terrified. My guy, Norb—we've been together thirteen years—lives and works part-time in Los Angeles, and my daughter, Darlene, lives in Laguna Beach. Cambria is a half-day drive for both. I want so badly for them to be with me, but I begin to worry about the upheaval I may soon cause in their lives. Tears flood my cheeks.

My bed is by the window. The warmth from the sun's reflection on the glass lessens the shivers pulsating through my body, although, oddly enough, I do not feel cold. The beautiful Santa Lucia mountain range is visible. Puffy white clouds hover over the mountains under a bright spring sky. The limbs of a young California oak tree sway in a gentle wind. The heaving stops. A thoughtful nurse provides another warm blanket. I draw it up under my chin to cover my arms and shoulders. It comforts me greatly, and I have the urge to hug the nurse for her kindness.

"Thank you," I say instead as she adjusts my pillow.

"Keep it under your head and neck but not your shoulders," she advises. I immediately notice the difference and feel foolish that it took me seventy-three years to learn this. Not too late, I hope. Well, I am alive and safe and warm...at this moment. And isn't this the only way we experience life, moment by moment?

My fear begins to subside as I think back on some of my most memorable moments and how grateful I am for them: I know what a warm summer breeze and a lover's tender kiss feel like on my cheek. I can recall the sound of waves breaking on the rocky shore just steps from my seaside cottage and the furious cries of my children and grandchildren as they responded to the slap that forced them to take that first breath. I took such pleasure in watching them grow, loving them, and being loved by them.

"I like living! I have sometimes been wildly, despairingly, acutely, miserably racked with sorrow, but through it all I still know quite certainly that just to be alive is a grand thing." Agatha Christie wrote these words, and I have lived them. Like so many, I have had my share of pain and sadness. But there are also many years of wonderful memories tucked away safely in the corners of my mind. Memories that are mine to recall and cherish until that very last breath. Some people have not been as fortunate.

I think about others battling cancer, especially children. Thousands of them are stricken every year. We've seen the images of young, hairless victims in hospital beds smiling bravely, their thin little arms reaching for cuddly stuffed animals offered to comfort them as this warm blanket does me. How unfair it is for them to be facing death before they have had a chance to experience the joy of living. The greatest tragedy of life is that not everyone gets a chance to grow old.

I think of my own first child, lost in a car accident more than thirty-five years ago when she was only eighteen. Debbie had just been crowned Homecoming Queen of Pasadena City College, and the very last photo I have of her was taken at that event by an *L.A. Times* photographer. She looked radiant, smiling and waving from the top of an open convertible as it made its way across the football field. A jeweled crown topped her long blonde hair, and a bouquet of roses lay tucked in her arm. As a final photo, it brings bittersweet memories. Sadly, it was not published to commemorate the homecoming event but to accompany the story of the accident a week later. "Homecoming Queen in Serious Condition," the headline blared, a chilling reminder that good news rarely takes precedence over bad.

But when I think of Debbie now, I smile, because I vowed long ago that I would never allow the tragedy of her early death to overshadow the wondrous joy that she brought to my life; it would be an injustice to always remember her through a flood of tears. Accidental death at such a young age *is* a tragedy. A body succumbing to cancer at seventy-three is, well, it's the natural order of things, like rose petals falling to the ground as summer ends. Sad, but expected and only temporary, until spring when a new generation bursts into bloom.

It's twilight now, and the room is drenched in shadow. My eyelids are heavy. I struggle against tears as I wonder at the conflicting emotions churning up inside me: melancholy mingled with gratitude; denial one minute that this is real and acceptance the next that my life may soon be over; optimism—*I can beat this*—mixed with quiet resignation—*I'm facing impossible odds*; anxiety over what happens tomorrow, followed by elation as I reflect on all my incredible yesterdays. Some feelings of regret gnaw their way to the surface. (Harold's pancakes?) But they are squashed by the pride I feel in knowing that I have also done some good along the way.

I'm confident these conflicts will resolve themselves...in time. I can only hope that when the final curtain draws to a close on my life, I will take that last bow with a wink, a wave, and a wily grin.

CHAPTER 3

You Can't Shop if You're Dead!

Darlene arrived at the hospital the next morning. We had barely exchanged hugs when Dr. Meiselman entered the room. I introduced them. His smile was warm and his handshake lingering. He took a deep breath and looked me straight in the eye as he began to explain, in great detail, the seriousness of the situation.

He spoke in even tones and said, "Indications are that the tumor might be in the head of the pancreas, an inoperable location." He paused slightly in anticipation of a response from me. None came.

"I'm also concerned that the cancer might have metastasized, as there is some kind of liquid floating around in the stomach, although, there's a chance it may be blood. But we can't do anything to address those issues yet because you've developed pneumonia from the vomiting."

Another pause. "There is also some internal bleeding, and we've discovered an infection on the esophagus."

Darlene and I glanced at each other. She sat stiffly, as though the slightest move, even to take a breath, might cause her to break down. My heart ached for her. I wanted to assure her that I would beat this thing, but the doctor's uneasy voice interrupted my thoughts.

"We'll have to address these issues and run a few more tests, so, unfortunately, cancer treatment will have to take a back seat until we eliminate these other problems," he continued.

Well, I didn't see that coming. My mind was still focused on *it may be in an inoperable position*. He then added that he would be leaving town for a few days. I wasn't sure what impact that would have on my treatment, but, hoping to lighten the mood, I looked him squarely in the eye and said, "Oooookay, then," in my best *Fargo* accent. His brows narrowed, indicating either that he had not seen the movie or was perplexed at my cavalier response. But I did get a smile out of Darlene.

The doctor began to inch his way toward the door when fear of uncertainty finally kicked in, and I asked him bluntly, "Any chance I could beat this?"

He hesitated a moment, then shook his head from side to side and said, "In all honesty, it would be tough."

"Doctor," I pressed, in another attempt to lighten things up, "if you're holding back any good news, now would be the time to let us have it." My second attempt at humor brought a hint of a smile to his wary face. "Just pray for blood," he said, before closing the door behind him.

Abandoning all hope of encouragement from the doctor, I murmured, "Go, me" under my breath. That would have to do for now.

Darlene could not remember Dr. Meiselman's name, so she called him something similar, "Nice Old Man," even though he wasn't old, and that's how we referred to him from then on.

Our little secret kept us in stitches every time the doctor entered the room, but he was never the wiser. Don't get me wrong, I had the utmost respect and admiration for all of the doctors and nurses, who, undoubtedly, are dedicated to saving lives, and I was so grateful to them. But hadn't I heard somewhere that laughter is the best medicine? I had to remember that!

I was facing that sonogram test on Monday to determine if the substance in my stomach was cancer cells or blood. I thought about the last thing Dr. Nice Old Man said before leaving: "Pray for blood!"

He, indeed, was a nice old man, and when the test two days later revealed that it *had* been blood and not rogue cancer cells, I couldn't wait to share the good news with him when he returned from...*Where?* I wondered. *A fishing trip, Vegas, or perhaps a conference*

*unveiling stunning new treatments raising the surviv-
ability rates for pancreatic cancer?*

Well, there was still the tumor to think about. How
long before I would know what stage it had reached
and if it was even operable? I let out a long sigh and,
drawing on the wisdom of Scarlett O'Hara in *Gone
with The Wind*, said to myself, *I won't think about
that now. I'll think about that tomorrow!*

A young hospital volunteer entered my room that
evening offering me a copy of *The Tribune*, a local
newspaper. I noticed an ad on page six announcing
that Williams Sonoma, my favorite gourmet cook-
ware store, was planning to open a branch in San Luis
Obispo early next year. *Damn,* I thought, as I began
to drift off into a deep sleep. *And I might not live long
enough to shop there!*

CHAPTER 4

A Virgo With a Plan, or Is That Redundant?

I spent the next six days in the hospital recovering from the complications I'd experienced after the initial test, and by then concerns had risen among friends in the small, close-knit community where I live.

Cambria is a charming town on the central coast of California, equidistant from Los Angeles and San Francisco. Uniquely nestled on hilly terrain between forested pine trees and the ocean, it boasts no chain stores nor a movie theater, but it hosts numerous art galleries, antique stores, fine restaurants, and cozy coffee houses.

I had been leading dance-aerobics and weight-training sessions three days a week at our local community center for about six years. There are more than seventy people on my list of participants, and, as they are a caring bunch, all were anxious for the latest news on my condition. To keep emails and phone calls to one another at a minimum, I decided I would communicate with the group via email with periodic updates. I thought it would also be a good way to keep other friends and out-of-town relatives up to date on my treatment and progress, but more importantly, to minimize any anxiety that my recovery might be, well, as is so often thought of with a diagnosis of pancreatic cancer...hopeless. Here's the first, sent on the day I returned home.

▶ EMAIL UPDATE: May 23, 2016

Okay, here's the scoop. You've probably heard I went into the medical center for a test last Tuesday, and as luck would have it, they had a ton of bed openings in the hospital. So, the doc came up with this crazy diagnosis of PC (no, not "politically correct," which I'm often accused of not being) but Pancreatic Cancer, and, bingo they soon waved an "admittance" form in my face. When he told me that there was a nasty tumor making a home in my pancreas I said "no way," but he stomped his foot and said, "Who's the doctor here?" He had a point, so, I gave in and signed on the dotted line. After all, a free bed and room service for a week I might like. The cancer...not so much.

There were four or five other complications after admittance, i.e. internal bleeding, pneumonia, an esophageal infection and, surprise, surprise, really high blood pressure, so they ordered a blood transfusion ($$$), antibiotics ($$), an oxygen machine ($$), and numerous other meds ($$$). Be careful the next time you check into a place; the extras can really add up. And, there wasn't a mini-bar in sight!

Anyway, I'm not telling you this for sympathy (although who could blame me?) but because there is a valuable lesson here. The hospital staff doctor who checked on me regularly looked at me grimly on Friday, the fourth day in the hospital, and told me it would take quite a few more days for me to get my strength back ($$$$) before I could start chemotherapy, but when he saw me on Monday, he said he was "astonished" at how quickly I'd improved and if nothing changed, he would send me home the next day.

I figured after six days of listening to the experts tell me how much they knew, I had some bragging rights of my own, so I said, "You know, Doctor, I teach aerobics and strength training three days a week so, other than the cancer thing, I think I'm in pretty good shape." His smile broadened and he nodded in agreement.

All right, you're thinking, "When is she going to get to the point?" But that is the point! I, we, are all in pretty good shape. So, on those days (and we all have them) that you want to sleep an extra hour or skip whatever exercise program you are on, DON'T DO IT! If/when something hits, the odds of recovery are far greater for those in good physical condition.

Rumor has it...

I know you want to know about my progress but rather than all of you asking one another, "How's Maryann doing?" and then some of you having Tuesday's latest, others Thursday's info, yada, yada, yada, I've devised a plan. Stop rolling your eyes. You all know I'm a Virgo! You give me a birthday present every year. In August. The last day. Only three short months from now.

So, here's the plan. When there's anything new, I will let you know and I promise, in a much briefer email than this one. If I'm otherwise occupied (like in surgery or something) then Diane C has agreed to do it.

Okay...the latest. I was released from the hospital this morning. I've been given referrals to an oncologist and a surgeon and advised to book appointments with them as soon as possible to begin chemotherapy and to determine if surgery is an option. (I sure hope I get to weigh in on that decision!)

Norb and my daughter (an ex nurse) are already actively involved in interviewing, er, researching the best possible hospitals outside the area. So far, City of Hope and Cedars (where Darlene once worked) seem the most promising, but UCLA and Stanford are also on the list.

So, here's what I have to do today: book a pedicure, book a haircut, book a massage, book the surgeon, book the oncologist...wait, scratch that! Book the oncologist, book the surgeon, book a pedicure and a haircut, and hope I have enough energy left to schedule a massage. In the meantime, thank you all, dear friends, for your concern and offers of help. It truly means a lot. But not to worry, I am going to beat this. Life is Good!

CHAPTER 5

Fishnet Stockings

They say it's the little things in life that get you down. I hate to argue with that logic, primarily because I don't know who "they" are or where to find them or how they define "little." "They" could be right, but the words of Dr. Andrew J. Galambos, a brilliant professor I once took courses from, also come to mind. He claimed that "most people are wrong about most things most of the time." Well, I'm not certain, but maybe I can cope with the big things, like pancreatic cancer, because I don't sweat the small stuff. So, when something minor hits—like when my favorite red nail polish is *brutally* yanked from the market without warning or the slightest concern over the dire consequences it might have on the loyal customer who has been using it for years and who, by the way (sniff), may soon be losing all of her hair—I tend to shrug it off.

Or not!

▶ EMAIL UPDATE: May 28, 2016

I went for that pedicure this morning and discovered that Essie is discontinuing "Fishnet Stockings," my favorite red nail polish. Honestly? Coping with cancer and having to find a replacement red at the same time! I hate when that happens! When Norb first saw that vivid and daring display of color on me a few years ago, he nicknamed me, "Toes." It's "Hi, Toes" and "Bye, Toes" and "let me help with the dishes, Toes" and "I love you, Toes." Losing the color is one thing, but will I lose an endearing nickname if I settle for a color with less of a "wow" factor?

On the good news side...I met my oncologist, Dr. Di-Carlo, and I LOVE him. He's a young, handsome, Italian fellow from the same neighborhood in Long Island that my family is from. He resembles and sounds like all my male relatives...Vinnie, Johnny, Frankie, Joey, Tony, Stevie, Ricky, and Bobby. (Oops, the last one's a female)

Plus, he's sharp and, in Norb's words, "new-age" when it comes to treatment. He is heavily involved in bringing clinical trials to the Central Coast but that's for future discussion. He believes that I am at stage 2 or 2½, an early stage, allowing for a more favorable outcome after treatment. However, he is ordering a PET scan to be sure. At this point, no one is certain the tumor is even operable, but chemotherapy should shrink it, making surgery—something he referred to as the Whipple procedure—more of an option. He convinced me. So, it looks like I'll start chemo next week for three months. If all goes well, surgery will follow sometime in August at UCLA, where they have an entire pancreatic unit. Woohoo! I may have to become a Bruins fan. (That's football, isn't it?)

Speaking of stages, I had to drop out of the production of The Dixie Swim Club after learning all of the dialog in scenes 1 thru 3 and half of scene 4. I know, right? But, I still have a leading role in "Love Letters" in October and I'm hoping to make that performance. I should be on the mend from surgery and I don't start chemo again until the first week in December. I might even have some hair by then!

Now, if only I could find a replacement for Fishnet Stockings.

CHAPTER 6

Doctor Doom: The Musical

Don't think *Fiddler on the Roof* and Tevye clicking his heels in the air in a celebration-of-life song or *Chorus Line* where you can delight in a series of quick kick-ball changes performed to the cheerful tune of "I Can Do That, I Can Do That."

No! Think *Phantom of the Opera's* dark dungeon and the mournful sounds of "Music of the Night" or *Sweeny Todd's* "The Best Pies in London," which is a pretty upbeat tune...until you find out that human flesh is baked into the pies. This sets the stage for my visit with Doctor Doom.

Okay. I may be exaggerating...just a little. I'll put it this way. It was certainly no *Walk in the Woods*. It left me with little hope that "The Sun Will Come Out Tomorrow." But "Don't Cry for Me" just yet.

Even though Dr. DiCarlo mentioned UCLA as a potential hospital for surgery, I followed up with a local surgeon I was referred to. Dr. Doom (not his real name) has an excellent reputation but performs pancreatic operations infrequently compared with UCLA, where they are performed daily, so I was leaning in that direction.

Norb was out of town, so my good friend Jeannie accompanied me to the appointment. We were sitting quietly in the office, thumbing through magazines, when Dr. Doom burst into the room smiling broadly and introducing himself with such flair that I thought he would burst into song. I figured he had seen my X-rays and just couldn't wait to tell me that the tumor was this tiny little thing, certainly revisable, and that I would live a long and healthy life once he cut the bloody thing out of my stomach. Wrong!

Still smiling, he waved the X-ray in front of us and talked about "all the dark spots" that he was "curious" about: one near the liver *(Whaaat?)*, and a few others that he ceremoniously pointed to. I began to wonder if he was in the wrong room.

He went on to say that if the tumor was at the head of the pancreas, an operation would not be possible because too many other things run through it, but if it was in the tail, there was a better chance of removing it *(Yes, I'd been told that)*. He indicated that he didn't think the Whipple operation—the procedure used to operate on pancreatic cancer patients—was an option for me.

I looked at Jeannie, who sat stunned, as I had led

her to believe that my chances were pretty good, and now we were hearing it's a game of—heads you lose, tails you may still lose!

"Have you seen the CAT scan?" Dr. Doom asked with more enthusiasm than I felt was appropriate. It was as though he were about to give me my first glimpse of an unborn child.

"No," I responded softly, wondering what difference it would make given this dismal news.

"Well, come on," he said as he grabbed my arm and led me out of the office and into a darkened room, where he promptly proceeded to pull up the scan on a computer screen. Jeannie wisely stayed behind, and I wished I'd had the courage to refuse the offer, too, but felt compelled to see this through. He pointed here and there and back again to light and dark shadows, and I followed his finger but found it hard to concentrate. I could not wrap my mind around the news of all the dark spots and the comment that he didn't think the Whipple procedure was an option.

When the theatrics were over, Dr. Doom marched me back into the room, where, still smiling and waving his arms, he went into a speech about how much progress has been made with pancreatic cancer patients.

"Life expectancy is now up to a year for many patients," he declared, failing to notice the gape in my mouth.

"But I've heard more favorable reports," I said questioningly.

"Yes, sometimes as much as two years," he quickly responded.

Jeannie and I looked at each other with a "Let's get the hell out of here" expression on our faces. His lips kept moving, but I tuned him out, and when the lips finally stopped, we hurriedly grabbed our belongings and rushed toward the door.

"I am going to order a PET scan so we can have a closer look; now let me give you a hug," he said as he thrust his arms around my shoulders. I stood stiffly for a moment, and when he let go, I slipped a forced smile in his direction. Outside the building, Jeannie asked, "What was all that about? I thought you felt your prospects for beating this were fairly good?"

"True," I answered. "But apparently, no one told Dr. Doom."

Maybe I was judging him too harshly. After all, his reputation in the community was stellar, and perhaps he thought his friendly manner would put me at ease. Or maybe I just didn't want to hear the truth. Either way, I decided I would ignore his instructions to call next week for the results of the PET scan and focus on Dr. DiCarlo's more optimistic opinion and my prospects with pancreatic specialists at UCLA.

Jeannie and I began to laugh the whole thing off as we arm-pointed and hip-swayed our way through the parking lot, singing, "Staying alive, staying alive, oh, oh, oh, oh, staying alive!"

I was not going to surrender so easily.

CHAPTER 7

Ode to
"The Californians"

Who doesn't love "Saturday Night Live's" popular skit "The Californians," which mocks our obsession to detail the specific street and freeway route taken on any given trip, to virtually anyone who will listen? (And that would be everyone, because we all do the same thing.) Did Norb and I discuss the most efficient route to the oncology center? Of course, we did. Did we tell our friends about it later? Totally! But New Yorkers making fun of Californians? Give me a break, dude! This update describes that visit.

▶ **E-MAIL UPDATE: JUNE 9, 2016**

Norb and I made our first trip to the Infusion Center yesterday for pre-chemo orientation. Took

Highway 1 to the railroad station, thinking we'd make a right and hit Broad, but the road curved around a bit throwing us off the track (no pun intended) to South Street which, luckily, turns into Santa Barbara Boulevard. From there, we turned left on Broad, just past the Starbucks, and it was a straight shot to Tank Farm Road and the office of my adorable oncologist, where there was lots of off-street parking.

After the administrative nurse formally introduced me to my first line of defense, "Mr." Gemzar, the cell-weakening drug and then "Mr." Abraxane, the heavy-hitting take-no-prisoners-alive, cell-bashing drug, she told me that my PET scan results were "negative." Well, I associate "negative' with things like "negative bank balance" (not so good) or as in captain to co-pilot, "Is the landing gear down?" "uh, Negative." (even worse.) So, I asked, judging by the look on the nurse's face, a really stupid question. "What does that mean?" I should have realized when Norb leaped out of his chair so fast he nearly hit the ceiling that this was a good thing. Still...as he literally jumped for joy, I waited for confirmation that his exuberance was justified. The nurse explained it to me but I can't spell "metastasizing" so I'll put it this way...the cancer HAS NOT SPREAD! Best news ever, right?

Not so fast! The nurse continued with a list of suggested "don'ts" while undergoing chemotherapy.

- Don't get an infection
- Don't lose weight
- Don't be around cats and kids
- Don't get mouth sores
- Don't have your teeth cleaned
- Don't have sex
- Don't ....

Wait, what?

Okay, fine! But I just found out Essie is replacing Fishnet Stockings with something called "Blushworthy." Sounds promising, but given the above, it may be a while before I can test it out on Norb.

CHAPTER 8

Meatballs and Helicopter Moms

Prior to my first treatment, several dear friends visited me to share their own experiences with chemotherapy so I would know what to expect. Dr. DiCarlo's plan called for three weeks on chemo and one week off for three months before surgery. The same protocol would be repeated after surgery. I was advised to have a "port" inserted under the skin of my chest to avoid being stuck with a needle every time the chemo was administered. This implant is done as an outpatient procedure at the local hospital. The port was good advice as I have small veins and it would have been painful and problematic to have so many infusions using the needle method. (I've had several instances in the past where frustrated nurses gave up and called for help.) The procedure was considered a minor operation, but I would have to face that dreaded nausea-inducing anesthesia again. Still, it would probably be worth it.

However, as luck would have it, I developed a high fever the day after the operation, and the doctor immediately ordered me back to the emergency center for treatment. Redness around the area made it obvious that the port had become infected. I had already broken one of the rules (*absolutely* do not get an infection) before treatment had even begun.

Thankfully, Darlene was with me that day, and her nursing background was a great comfort. Given that it's a forty-minute drive to the hospital and my temperature continued to rise, I started to panic, but she remained calm and reassuring.

Darlene studied nursing after high school, ultimately working at two of the finest hospitals in Southern California: Pasadena Memorial and Cedars Sinai. But when she married and started a family, *they* became her priority, and she quit nursing to give them her full attention. I have never known a more patient and loving mother. I guess they are referred to as "helicopter moms" now because they seemingly hover over their children. Perhaps that's a good thing. When I see the results in my grandchildren, Taylor and Chase, I applaud her. But her story doesn't stop there.

When the kids grew and became involved in activities outside the home, Darlene decided to pursue one of her long-time interests—photography—and went back to school to study the craft. Now she runs her own successful photo business focusing on architecture and working primarily with property developers in the Laguna Beach area. I worried, as she made several trips to Cambria to care for me, that as an independent business owner she was taking too much time away from her clients to "hover" over me. Helicopter daughter?

Darlene has a very keen sense of life, and it shows in her images. Photography is an art, and art is a re-creation of reality. How one sees life, I believe, is reflected in one's daily work. Her images capture the human mind's ability to create structures that are functional and enduring but also stunningly beautiful, a tribute to the architects who design them.

I had been looking through copies of *Dwell* and other prestigious magazines containing her photos when she noticed my port scar was turning bright red, indicating it might be infected. I soon felt my temperature rising, and that's when we called the doctor.

When we arrived at the hospital, the emergency room was packed and we waited four hours before being admitted to an examining room. They had been holding out for a private room to keep me away from "potentially infectious" other patients. (Had they seen the waiting room??) Dar asked for a mask to at least cover my nose and mouth, as folks were coughing and sneezing all over the place and my temperature was approaching 104. Once inside the exam room, it took three more hours for tests and a prescription for antibiotics. Then we finally made our way back home.

Darlene had been making turkey meatballs for

our dinner, and when we left for the hospital in a hurry, she'd abandoned them on the stove. Upon our return nine hours later, Dar didn't think it was safe to eat them.

"I think they'll be fine," I said, but she trashed them anyway.

"Mom," she replied, "they've been sitting out all day. I'll just make a new batch." The image of her as she patiently and lovingly began to measure and pour the ingredients into a bowl will forever be etched in my mind. Not because the meatballs were so delicious (they were) but for what it said about my "hovering" daughter. One does not always need a camera to capture an enduring moment in time.

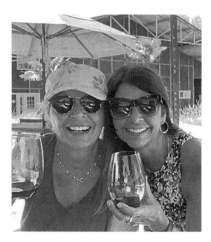

With my daughter, Darlene

CHAPTER 9

The Oncology Center

Norb arrived a few days later and accompanied me to the oncology center for that first treatment. He could tell I was nervous and tried to allay any anxiety, but nothing could have prepared me for what I was about to see.

After we checked in at the reception desk, a nurse came for me and walked me back to the two large treatment rooms opposite each other. Each room contained approximately ten recliner chairs, and all but one was occupied with men and women of all ages, sizes, shapes, colors, and stages of decline. A chilling scene. I remember thinking, *I do not belong here.* Tears began to well in my eyes, but the nurse's call to "jump up on that scale and let's get your weight" was enough of a distraction to allow me to regain my composure.

"One twenty-four. Is that your normal weight?

Normal? "Yes, normal," I replied, wondering if things would ever be normal again.

Most patients were elderly and frail but not all of them. Some months later, I discovered a smaller room in the rear of the facility reserved for children. A few patients slept, some read, others talked softly with friends or family. Sadness reflected in the eyes of some, a trace of hope in others, and resignation in most, as though this was part of some grand scheme—expected and inevitable and, in any case, out of their control.

A few of the patients aimed weak smiles in my direction. My heart ached for them and their predicament, as though I wasn't facing initiation into the same club. The question *Why me?* flashed through my mind followed immediately with the obvious answer... *Why not me!*

Every lounger had a small chair next to it for family or friends who brought the patients in. I settled into an empty lounger beside a window, then accepted a pillow and warm blanket and pressed them to my face. Softness. Warmth. I know this. This is familiar. It's going to be okay. Norb plunked himself into a chair beside me and squeezed my hand.

The other room had no windows, and over the following months, I suffered enormous anxiety upon entering the center before each treatment, afraid I might land in that darker room. Ignoring, at great peril, one of the less offensive Commandments—the one about coveting thy neighbor's property—I coveted the window seat and glared angrily at any poor wretched soul who might have reached it before me.

I wanted to look outside of that room for the next three hours to glimpse—if only a narrow slice of it—the world where everything existed as it should. I sighed with relief each time I secured a seat in the room with the window and, the Tenth Commandment be damned, suffered burning envy on the rare instance that I did not.

Of course, when I reflect back, I regret those feelings. But who would argue that an amendment to The Tenth isn't called for? Clearly, the author was running out of transgressions, and this, being the last, could be considered by any stretch of the imagination as...a rounding error. Ten sounds well-thought-out. Nine, not so much. A looser interpretation could go something like this: "Thou shalt not let greed or jealousy cause you to covet thy neighbor's property...unless you're really, really sick, in which case, barring any more serious transgressions, all might be forgiven."

Nurse Kathy was warm and friendly, as was every nurse that administered my treatment over the next six months. She explained the procedure: A saline solution first. Then the drug Gemzar, followed by the Abraxane. Bags were hung on an IV stand behind the chair. A needle containing the saline solution to clean the port was quickly inserted, causing a brief burning sensation and some nausea. Thus, the three-hour "drip" began.

Once the saline solution drained, the Gemzar would slowly snake its way through the tube and, with any luck, directly target the cancerous growth latching itself to my weakening pancreas. When the Gemzar bag was empty, a buzzer would go off and the nurse closest to me would quickly replace it with a full bag of the Abraxane, but not before asking me, again, my name and birthdate—a commitment to safety that was impressive and greatly appreciated.

Patients would come and go, all in various stages of treatment and, by their appearance, stages of cancer. Soon, snacks would be passed around by the nurses: coffee, tea, water, chips, and crackers. Eating during the procedure was encouraged as it helped with the nausea and also passed the time. A bell lay on the small table attached to the lounger in case of an emergency, but the nurses were always so close and attentive that the slightest moan would have brought several of them running in seconds. Bags were changed periodically but, again, not before asking my name and birthdate.

Norb and I would read, eat lunch, and check emails to pass the time. I never slept. There was no time to waste on sleep; that would have felt like I was losing control, giving up, letting go. The lunch Norb brought for us always included health-food bars or boxes of chocolate for the nurses. His light banter also brought a cheeriness to the room that matched the mood these dedicated nurses—being the closest things on earth to angels—tried their best to create and sustain.

On weeks that Norb was not in town, other friends accompanied me. We would play cards, talk about shopping (Williams Sonoma should be opening soon), the day's news, the weather, and, of course, the best route to take home. Anything to get my mind off the poison being fed into my system, drop by drop. I kept telling myself, *it is destroying the cancer and will save my life*! But I wasn't always convinced.

Darlene and I went to a movie following one treatment. It was the debut of "Absolutely Fabulous," or "Ab Fab," as the hit TV series was called in Britain. It was my favorite program, and I watched it regularly for the five years that I lived in London. A comedy was just what I needed, and seeing Jennifer Saunders and Joanna Lumley in the roles they made famous made me feel like I was reunited with old friends. And for a little while, things seemed normal again.

The negative effects of chemo usually hit twenty-four to thirty-six hours after the treatment, so following the movie, we were able to enjoy dinner at Giuseppe's, my favorite Italian restaurant, with even a little sip of wine. But, the chemo was infused with energy-producing steroids for quicker absorption, so a day or two later, my body always received conflicting messages. Half of me whined, "This is shitty, I feel like I'm dying," and the other half shouted back, "I get it, but let's run the 10K in the meantime!"

The cumulative effect of chemo took its toll on me a few months later. Some days I was barely able to stand on my own. So Norb devised a little game to help me out of bed or off the couch. "Stay flat," he urged me as he leaned over me, took my arms, and wrapped them around his neck. "Hang on tight," he'd say. Then as he stood up, my rag-doll of a body would rise with him without expending any energy or effort on my part.

We laughed and laughed at that routine every time, and I didn't mind at all feeling like a child again.

CHAPTER 10

Little Green What?

I have to admit I was overwhelmed by all the pills I had to take throughout my treatment: Fluconazole, Gluconase, Ducolax, Ducosate, Compazine, Cephalexin Voltaren, Imodium, Bisacody, Probiotics, Turmeric, Hydrocodone-acetaminophen, Diyclomine, Miralax, Pantoprazole, Promethazine, Benzonatate, Nystatin, Prochlorperazine, Lorazepam, and Ondansetron among them.

There were days I stood looking at that pile of crap and thought, *just shoot me now.*

I couldn't remember what to take at what time or what it was for. I had to keep reading the labels, which was frustrating, time-consuming, and required a search for my glasses every time. As usual, Norb came to the rescue. First, he labeled the top of each bottle with a black marker in easily recognizable terms such as nausea, cough, sleep, pain, thrush, cramps, enzymes, turmeric, B12, and so on. That stopped the cursing and crying at pill time.

But the bottles were spread all over my kitchen table and looked a mess when anyone came to visit, so I decided to put them in a compartmentalized sock box I took from my dresser drawer. The French blue-and-white flowered fabric almost looked decorative on the table; all the tops could be read and the bottles easily removed. When guests were due, I just picked the box up and hid it in another room. I had to show Norb I wasn't totally bereft of ideas. But he soon out-did me...again.

He insisted I start a diary to record—by day and time—every pill I took and every bite of food I ate, along with any reactions I might have experienced, in an easy-to-read, three-column format.

"Easier to monitor any adverse reactions," he said.

That worked out well for a while. I listed gluco-nase, compazine, turmeric, and the others under the "meds" column dutifully for a few weeks. Then, to save time, I started to abbreviate: glu, comp, tur, but eventually I got bored and just wrote S.O.S.—"same old shit"—in that column each day unless something changed.

I was advised to eat five small meals a day, but the nausea left me with no appetite, so three snack-type meals was all I could manage. I kept my food intake simple and repetitive, so that column was easy. Scone at 8:00 a.m., yogurt at noon, and soup at 6:00 p.m.

Then, the "little green cookies" came into my life. A very close friend brought them over one day.

For nausea, she said.

Uh, I've never...

Just try 'em. They'll help with pain, too.

But, what if...

They won't harm you. Trust me.

But it's against the law, I said, thinking I'd come up with a good excuse.

Not for medical purposes, she said, smiling.

Oh, what the hell, if it stops the nausea, I thought. *Don't be such a sissy*. Cautiously, I took about one-quarter of the "cookie" and sampled it. Hmmm. Tasty. A while later, my nausea disappeared. Cool!

The next day I took a little bit more, about half. I became increasingly curious to discover what all the fuss was about. Tried three-quarters the following day. Nice, no nausea but not much else. That's okay. I was fearful as a "newbie" that I'd have a bad reaction. But on the fourth day, I mustered up a bit of courage and tried a whole one...strictly for experimental purposes, you understand. Here's that day's food column entry:

8:00   Green cookie
9:00   Scone and coffee
9:30   Scrambled eggs
10:00 Toast and jam
10:30 Granola, yogurt, nuts, cranberries

11:00 Wobbling toward the fridge... *Uh, is it lunch time yet?*

11:30 Turkey Sandwich with chips

12:30 Ice cream

1:30 Checking the clock, *Shouldn't I be having a snack about now?*

It went on like that all day until my sleepy little head hit the pillow, but not before warning myself to stick to the one-quarter portion.

The next day, I called Darlene to tell her about the ordeal. My twenty-two-year old grandson, Chase, could overhear the conversation, and they both broke into hysterical laughter.

"Sure, make fun of grandma," I warned. "My friend promised that the next batch will be chocolate...and I don't share!"

CHAPTER 11

Ali's Artichoke Ravioli...and More

Residing in this kind and caring community almost made me forget that I'm living with a life-threatening disease. Almost. As expected, the debilitating effects of chemo left me with neither the energy nor the desire to do much cooking, although with the nausea issue resolved, thanks to the little green cookies, my appetite was improving. And there was a well-organized plan among my friends and neighbors to keep me well-fed while going through the treatments. Nourishing home-cooked meals—beef bourguignon, lamb tagine, artichoke ravioli, Irish stew, bone broth, deviled eggs, chicken soup, and much more—were delivered to me on a daily basis. Ali's artichoke ravioli was one of my favorites.

All the meals were made "freezable" so I could use

them when needed. I must confess, I began to wonder how I could keep those wonderful dishes coming when I got better. And if I didn't...get better...then for Norb, who, when he was here, got to share in them. The guy is an eating machine! I made Di promise to set up a "Go Feed Me" page for him so he wouldn't starve after I was gone. At least for a little while.

I belong to a local group called Cambria Wine Divas. Each month, we visit a different winery (there are three hundred in the area) and enjoy a picnic lunch while tasting everything from rose to pinot to a variety of blends. After ten years of monthly visits, I could recite in my sleep the descriptions pourers used to point out the uniqueness of their own wines, and I drew on that experience for the update I sent out after the first round of chemo.

► EMAIL UPDATE: JULY 2, 2016

I'm not ashamed to admit that, at the moment, it really sucks to be me. Whoever is in charge of side effects went down the list and made sure I wasn't deprived of a single one of them. Nausea, check. Diarrhea, check. Constipation, check. Mouth sores, check. Chemical taste, muscle pain, bone pain, fever, check, check, check, and check.

Treatments for some of the side effects comes with—you guessed it—their own set of side effects. It's a real balancing act.

The most annoying side effect was the awful taste chemo left in my mouth. The particular combination of drugs I was taking—I'll call them the "Reserve" blend—were brimming with the complex flavor of chemicals like lead and iodine while delivering secondary notes of sulfur and the pungent taste of...rotten cheese. The "nose" was reminiscent of highly acidic cow pie with just a hint of freshly poured and still-steaming asphalt. The smoky aroma of hot tar makes an appearance as the "nose" lingers. None of these finish with the slightest silky, smooth taste of, say, melted chocolate. So, is it any wonder that I'm losing weight?

The good news is that I met with Dr. Donahue, the surgeon at UCLA, and he said he believed the tumor is "revisable." I wasn't familiar with that term but he was smiling so I figured it meant he could cut the damn thing out. Lucky me, because I discovered that only a mere 15 to 20 percent of pancreatic patients can be helped with surgery. The program called for two more rounds of chemo (two months) and then surgery at the Ronald Reagan Hospital at UCLA, followed by three more months of chemo (ugh). But, hey, with news like that, I say, bring it on, side effects and all.

CHAPTER 12

Chemo Buddy

Norb was my rock throughout chemo. He was always positive and upbeat and creative and playful and supportive and, and, and...I can't say enough about him. His physical and emotional strength kept me in check. And his sense of humor kept my spirits high.

One day while I was undergoing treatment at the oncology center, he blew up one of the nurses' blue rubber gloves, drew a face on it, and called it my "chemo buddy," someone to keep me company while he went out to get our lunch. The nurses adored Norb. They said nothing about the stolen glove or the childlike behavior.

There was nothing childlike, though, about our first date fourteen years ago. We met in a local coffee shop one morning and became fast friends, but I resisted broadening our relationship when he asked me out. After several months of asking, he wore me down, and I agreed to only one date—dinner at a favorite Italian restaurant. I showed up with a list of reasons why I could not see a future for us, and I went through them one by one throughout the meal. Top of the list was our age difference. I will admit to being ten years older but nothing more. (Okay, twelve or so.) I'd been twice widowed; he had never been married. I had grown children and a huge family; he had only his mother. My job had me traveling frequently; he owned a small business that kept him pretty much local. I was into business suits and briefcases; he was into jeans and boots (which he wore well, by the way.) I was hoping these issues would be enough to discourage him. It wasn't. He argued every point, beginning with "age is just a number," until I was exhausted and we left.

Prior to our meeting the night of our first date, he asked me to park on the top level of the parking structure, about six stories off the ground. The thought occurred to me that he might be planning to throw me off the roof if I refused to see him again. But I was wrong. It was a warm summer evening, and the roof level provided a lovely view of the mountains surrounding Old Town Pasadena. When we reached his car, he opened the door, slipped a CD into the player, pressed "play," and when the music began, he grabbed me by the waist and began to dance me around the rooftop to Trisha Yearwood's "Little Hercules," a song about a strong-willed, independent woman who...well, you probably get the point. "We may never have another chance to do this," he said half smiling, half frowning as he whirled me around. Cars passed us, waving and beeping their horns. I had to admit it was pretty romantic, but still, I wasn't going to change my mind.

Well, some months later, as I was backing out of my garage, I noticed something swinging from the handle as the garage door creaked its way open. *What the heck?* I thought. I hopped out of the car, brought the door down, and grabbed the bag. Inside was a cup of coffee and my favorite cappuccino chocolate chip muffin from the local coffee shop where we met most mornings. *That's it! Differences be damned*, I thought, and later agreed to see a movie with him. He still brings me those muffins on his frequent trips to Cambria.

I wanted to take Chemo-Buddy to UCLA with me, but the little guy's air escaped over time, and he flattened out. I wasn't worried. Norb would be there... as always.

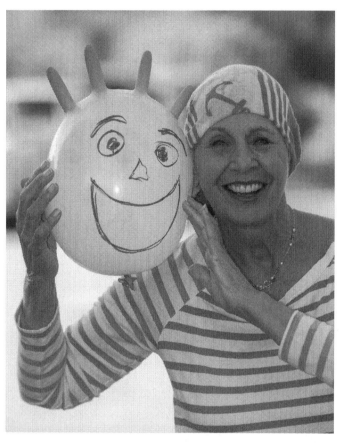

My Chemo Buddy

CHAPTER 13

Grandchildren: Life's Greatest Reward

Both of my grandchildren visited me during treatment. Chase, twenty-three at the time, was a sweet and gentle soul. When I stood next to him, his six-foot frame made me feel like I was the child and he the adult. We have always had a very special relationship. How many young men would spend ten days in a car with their grandmother touring Arizona, Texas, and New Mexico as Chase and I did just a few short months before I was diagnosed?

We listened to history books on tape and in between tapes, sang our way through his and my playlists of country-western favorites. We even visited Billy Bob's famous honky-tonk in Fort Worth, where I taught him some dance steps. A few of his high school friends who had moved to Texas met us there, but he wasn't at all embarrassed to be seen two-stepping around the dance floor with his grandmother. He was (is!) sooooo cool.

When Chase and Taylor visited, I did my best to appear as normal as possible. It wasn't hard to put on a cheery face, since my spirits were never higher than when I was around my grandchildren. I'm sure they took the cue from me as they behaved in a similar fashion. I sensed the "You've got this, Nan" attitude from both. If they had any fear that I might not survive, they hid it well. Apparently, my optimist gene worked its way into their blessed little hearts.

On one of the visits, I took Chase to a new brewery in the Paso Robles area called the Barrel House for some beer tasting. It reminded me of the time I took him to Whistler Resort in Canada for his high school graduation. "You know, Nan, in Canada you can drink at eighteen," he informed me after barely clearing customs in Vancouver. "I'm just sayin'," he added with a sly smile and a shrug of the shoulders. So, yes, we ordered a beer with dinner that night and toasted his coming of age.

That afternoon at the Barrel House he looked so grown up, and it saddened me a little. *Where did the years go?* I wondered. *And how many more would I have left to share in his future and get to know the family that he would someday have?* Well, it's the here and now that counts. We sat in the warm sunshine listening to a local band's version of an old Eagles tune.

The sound of water splashing in a nearby fountain added to the day's pleasure as we guzzled down the cool, locally crafted beer. Well, *he* guzzled. *I* sipped. Grandmothers don't guzzle.

Taylor, my darling twenty-six-year-old grand-daughter, visited too. Though it may not be too hard to imagine, Taylor chose Paris and London for her graduation trip, much to my delight. With my years in London, I was eager to show her the sights and take her to some of the many wonderful shows and museums the city had to offer. In Paris, we picnicked on the concrete banks of the Seine, nibbling cheese and sipping wine as the bells of Notre Dame rang out on the other side of the river.

On this recent visit to Cambria, we again shared wine and cheese, but this time in the little gazebo in my garden. No river, no church bells, but we could see a slice of ocean a few blocks away, and all my roses were in bloom. We talked about the documentary Taylor was working on (she has a degree in film production from Chapman U), which included filming some of the prison population at San Quentin who practice yoga. She's a tiny little thing, probably carrying no more than one hundred pounds on her five-foot-two-inch frame, but she travels the world hauling camera equipment and luggage in places that are not easy travel destinations: Peru, Cameroon, India, Norway, the Maldives, Dubai. As I write this, she is on her way to Uganda to film an annual fundraiser event for Action in Africa, a non-profit group helping to support education and healthcare needs for children and adults in the neediest communities. I worry about her when she's away. She's been instructed to call me the minute her feet hit the ground here at home after every trip, and I'm relieved that she is willing to indulge me by doing just that.

Out in the gazebo, Taylor tried on several of the sun hats and scarves I used to cover my naked head—a coy effort on her part, I began to think, to let me know I looked perfectly natural wearing the cancer regalia. I'd always felt when I was out and about with all those silly scarves that it was obvious my hair was gone.

Taylor took a few selfies of us and later posted them on Facebook. I got a few "likes." She got three marriage proposals.

Several weeks later, a package arrived from Taylor. Her work schedule was not going to allow her to visit me on my birthday, so she sent a present but marked the box in large, bold letters on all four sides: "Do not open till August 31st!" *Damn*, I thought. *Stare at that package for two weeks? The little brat! Well, two can play at that game.* I quickly dashed off an email to thank her and to let her know that...her Christmas present was on the way!

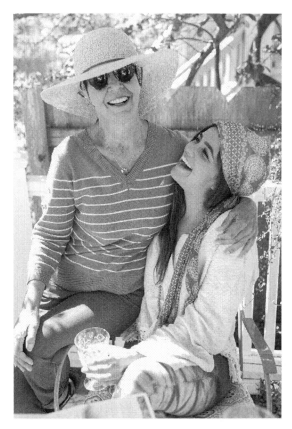

With my granddaughter, Taylor

CHAPTER 14

Stripes or Checks?

As if I didn't already have enough to deal with—the chemo, finding a replacement for Fishnet Stockings, and all—I was awakened one night around 2:00 a.m. to the sound of rushing water. I slipped and slid my way into the kitchen, where something had broken under the sink. In my chemo-addled brain-state, I couldn't remember where the shutoff valve was, so, not wanting to keep all the excitement to myself, I called my neighbors—Bill and Di—who live across the street. They rushed over, found the valve, and turned it off.

We spent the rest of the night sweeping water out the front and back doors and wringing out towels in an attempt to dry the place up. "That wasn't the end," to quote Winston Churchill. "It wasn't even the beginning of the end. It was just the end of the beginning" of what turned out to be a major disaster. Here's the update I sent out a few days later.

▶ EMAIL UPDATE: AUGUST 18, 2016

This report is being filed from an undisclosed foreign location.

Well, okay, not "foreign," I'm actually just around the corner. The coffee's great, and there's a cat.

After the flood at 2 a.m. a few weeks ago that ruined my hardwood floor under which they discovered asbestos three layers down, I was forced to move out, literally, until some guys in plastic suits and hoods got rid of the stuff. Before they started, they taped yellow strips on the front door with the warning "Do Not Enter, Could Cause Cancer."

SERIOUSLY?

So, long story even longer, I was offered the use of a lovely guest house by my good friends Judy and Raimund while the whole mess was being cleaned up. After picking out new flooring and carpeting, (thankfully, my daughter arrived in town in time to help) I noticed my window treatment could use some updating and actually, I had been hunting for new fabric to recover a chair and sofa before I was diagnosed and ... well, doesn't everyone remodel while undergoing chemo?

You're probably asking yourself, "Could things get any worse?"

Well, yes, and they did. After the flood, Darlene and I had begun packing and loading two of every-thing in the ark—uh—car for my move out when I got word that some of my white blood cells had decided to hit the road (cowardly little bastards!) My "adorable Dr. D" quickly ordered a series of shots, which began producing replacement cells so, good riddance and who needs quitter cells anyway?

And then, AND THEN...

While at chemo today, Dr. DiCarlo came in to say that yesterday's CT scan showed the tumor had shrunk and I should be ready for surgery in about six weeks.

With any luck, that might just be enough time to find fabric that hasn't been "discontinued" ...like the last nine samples I ordered!

CHAPTER 15

How Can I Help?

I have always believed in the natural goodness of mankind, but never has this been more evident to me personally than hearing the following four words from friends and neighbors when my life was suddenly turned upside down: *How can I help?*

Norb's work schedule only allowed him to get to Cambria eight to ten days a month. Darlene was running her own photography business in Orange County, so for most of my treatment I was pretty much alone.

But I was never *on my own*.

It didn't take long for friends and neighbors to flood me with offers of help. I was absolutely blown away, to say the least. In addition to the cooked meals they brought to the house, they did so much more: they offered to grocery shop for me and they took turns driving me to doctor visits and chemo treatments (forty minutes each way and three hours for the treatment).

My good friends Di and Bill, who helped me in the middle of the night with the flood, were especially helpful. They hand-watered my garden. And Di volunteered to oversee the installation of carpeting and the finishing touches on the painting that had not been completed before I had to leave for UCLA and surgery. When I arrived home ten days later, everything was perfectly in place.

Several friends knitted me hats and scarves to keep my hairless head and neck warm. I was never without either.

Some of the girls in my dance/aerobics classes volunteered to spend endless hours putting together music and choreography so they could lead the sessions in my absence. They took turns covering for me for almost a year. I admit I sometimes worried that I might not be missed, but the vigorous round of applause, the whooping and hollering that greeted me on my first day back convinced me I need not have worried.

In addition to the guesthouse offer during asbestos cleanup, other friends helped with my gardening, trimming, cutting, weeding. Still others kept me entertained with card or board games, though it would have been nice if they had let me win a little more often.

Not a day went by when there weren't several get-well cards in the mail. Flowers and plants arrived. Mail and papers were carried up the driveway and placed squarely on the welcome mat at the front door.

The outpouring of kindness, generosity, and compassion in this tiny community was truly overwhelming.

One day, a small package from my granddaughter arrived, bringing a flood of tears to my eyes. Wrapped tightly to prevent breakage were three little bottles of...Fishnet Stockings! Two weeks later, several more bottles arrived from a dear niece living in San Diego.

I could only imagine the calls that must have gone out to beauty supply stores and nail salons all over Southern California to round up the last supply of that luscious red polish. I wonder if the run on that color ever gave Essie second thoughts about discontinuing it.

"I think I might have enough for a lifetime," I said as I handed the precious bottles to Christine, my manicurist, for safekeeping at my next appointment. I was afraid I might forget to bring one along to the salon every time I needed a pedicure.

Christine quickly shoved the bottles in the back of a small drawer on her manicure table, out of sight of other customers.

"No one in this town is going to wear Fishnet Stockings but Maryann," she giggled as she slid the drawer closed. "No one!"

CHAPTER 16

Hair Today, Gone Tomorrow

Wow! No hair, no brows, no lashes, no pride! I no longer wanted to look in the mirror. "Ugly" was the word that quickly came to mind. But Dr. DiCarlo had encouraged me to visit the near-by Hearst Cancer Resource Center on my first visit with him. The center, funded primarily by the Hearst Foundation, as well as community donations, provided information, support, nutritional advice, and other helpful services to cancer patients on a complimentary basis. They offered classes in meditation, music therapy, yoga and many others for patients and their caregivers.

One of the services included a makeup and wig session designed to help cover up sallow skin, sticky eyes, drawn cheeks, and a balding head. "If you look good, you'll feel good," was their philosophy. I had been putting on makeup for fifty-odd years and was a bit skeptical I could learn anything new. But I instinctively felt it would do me good to be with others that were perhaps having the same thought when looking in the mirror—*I look awful.* So, I signed up.

There were eight of us in the session and two volunteer instructors. We were given a bag of products generously donated by the cosmetic companies and then shown how to apply them to our best advantage. Most of us had already been through chemo, so our faces were pale or dry or blotchy, and the creams and cover-ups did make us look—and feel—better.

They also provided us with lovely long scarves and showed us how to wrap them around our heads in a variety of flattering ways. One style was to twist the ends of the scarf into the shape of a rose at the nape of the neck, but I couldn't get the hang of it and opted for a wig instead. Later, when Taylor brought me a scarf that she had tied in just such a manner, it became my favorite. When the weather changed and it got cold or rained, I opted for wool hats or baseball caps (the wigs were itchy), which were easier to put on and take off. It became obvious that I was bald, but by that time, I didn't care. My vanity goes only so far.

On that first visit, as the stylist began wrapping a scarf around the head of one of the women who hadn't lost her hair yet, the woman began to sob. I understood, because I did the same when my hairdresser, Sheila, shaved my head after my first few rounds of chemo. I was shedding hair all over the place; on my clothes, my pillow case, in the shower, my car, and I knew it was time. I think I cried more because Sheila refused to charge me for the shave. Her warmth and generosity at such a difficult time in my life was truly heartwarming. My manicurist, Christine (of Fishnet Stockings fame), offered to give me complimentary leg massages every week during cancer treatment. I couldn't possibly take advantage of that offer more than once. Okay, twice.

After the operation, I had to wait seven weeks before my second round of chemo, and my hair began to grow back. I knew I would lose it soon, and when it began to fall out, I wasted no time calling Sheila, who rendered me bald again. That time, as the shaver buzzed around, tickling my head and neck, I could not stop laughing.

Some months later when my hair began to grow back, it was thick and curly, unlike my normal thin and straight hair. A customer in the French Bakery looked at me admiringly one day and said, "I would die for hair like that."

Her mouth dropped open when I quickly replied, "I almost did."

CHAPTER 17

Legal Issues

Maybe I should have read some of those books on coping with cancer that Norb was thoughtful enough to get for me. Maybe I should have gone to one of those "safe-spaces" in Berkeley, hugged a bunny, and waited for the whole thing to blow over. That's the advantage of living in California; it's a reality-free zone. *No worries.*

But I was looking for a middle ground, and I found it. I decided to ignore all the gritty and frightening details in those books, put myself in the hands of the experts, follow their advice, and trust that all would be well. However, a little more knowledge might have saved me from an embarrassing moment with one of those experts.

▶ EMAIL UPDATE: SEPTEMBER 8, 2016

Breaking news: Tumor's Days Are Numbered

I spoke to the Nurse Practitioner/Legal Advisor at UCLA today and am happy to say my surgery is scheduled for Monday, September 19. I have to jump through a few hoops first—like lab tests, and an EKG to prove I'm a good candidate for surgery—but I should pass with flying colors, I hope, I hope, I hope.

First, of course, they insist you sign some legal documents that absolve them of pretty much everything should anything go wrong. In an operation they call the Whipple procedure, the surgeon is going to slice open the stomach of a seventy-three-year-old woman who has a history of missing body parts, remove the tail of the pancreas, the duodenum, a portion of the bile duct, maybe part of the stomach, and the spleen. Then, reconnect the remaining intestine, bile duct, and pancreas, stitch up all the loose stuff, and staple it all closed. What could go wrong?

But, rules are rules, so in fulfilling her duties to be sure I understood the procedure and the risk, Nurse Kratchett—er, Kathy—asked if I had any questions. Yes, fine on the tumor, I thought, but the spleen? I don't even know what a spleen is and what it does, but I thought I should express some allegiance to the body part that's probably served me well for seven decades. "So," I asked, "will the spleen be put back in?" I could swear her eyes rolled back in her head and after a long pause, she said, "Noooope." Not wanting to show any further ignorance on my part, I shook my head in under-standing and uttered this brilliant retort: "Uh huh!"

Now that's probably why they are so darned fussy about legal issues. Apparently, one doesn't need a spleen so I wouldn't have missed it and I'm not the kind who would sue over a non-significant body part anyway. Maybe I should have Googled it but it's too late now. I sheepishly signed the approval papers.

In other news:

Just when I'm beginning to appreciate how much money I'm saving on shampoo and hair-cuts, my hair is starting to grow back. Well, only about an eighth of an inch, standing straight up and prickly, but a welcome sight anyway. Although, with more chemo scheduled for after the operation, I'll soon be bald again. Sheila has offered to shave it when it begins to fall out, as she did after the first round of chemo. I'm pretty sure that this time, I won't cry.

Speaking of the theatre:

You may know that I'm appearing in Love Letters, a play directed by Nancy Green, at the Cambria Center for the Arts and Theatre, on October 28th, 29th and 30th. If you're planning to attend, it's not too early to mark your calendars. Hopefully, kinky hair and a missing spleen won't jeopardize my performance. But if it does, I'm pretty certain you can't sue me. I learned a few things at UCLA today.

P.S. In case you're wondering, the birthday present from Taylor (yes, I waited until the 31st to open it) contained a ton of turmeric, the most highly recommended cancer-fighting supplement. "Not a glamourous gift," the note read, "but promise you'll take these every day."

I take it back. She is NOT a brat!

CHAPTER 18

Bam! Zap! Kapow!

Forget Spiderman, Superman, and Wonder Woman with their silly, pseudo super powers. A white, sticky substance shooting out from a hand and you can wall-crawl! Really? A man of steel with the ability to leap tall buildings in a single bound? Bor-ing! And don't get me started on that skinny little wonder-bitch with the eighteen-inch waist. No! My Super Hero is Doctor Scott Donahue, Surgeon Extraordinaire.

I'm in the UCLA Operating room, September 19, 2016.

That last knockout drug has me drifting lazily in outer space, finger painting happy faces on passing cumulus clouds. My Super-Surgeon slips into his blue super-scrubs, dons a paper hat, squeezes his long, nimble fingers into plastic gloves, and ties a white mask around his face, leaving only intense blue eyes to reveal his true identity. My hero is ready! With deadly speed and precision, he whips out a razor-sharp scalpel, carves an s-shaped opening in my stomach, and, before you know it, Zap! That tumor is *terminated*!

Now, as I zoom through the galaxy at warp speed in search of something chocolate, he, without even breaking a sweat, scurries from one lymph node to another in search of hidden rogue cells, and Bam! The evil little monsters blast off for parts unknown. Then, while I'm happily performing delightful little loop-de-loops in search of distant galaxies, he takes a little stitch here and a little stitch there, and Kapow! Another life saved! Now that's what I call an extraordinary display of Super Powers!

With a sigh of self-satisfaction, my hero quickly removes his Super-Surgeon disguise and, undetected, slips back into the real world as mild-mannered Dr. Scott Donahue. Never mind that he leaves me behind for a game of hide-and-seek with the sun.

But I'm getting ahead of myself. The day didn't start that way.

———— * * * ————

I'd had some trepidation when I entered the hospital that morning. The hubbub reminded me of Grand Central Station—people scurrying everywhere; patients, visitors, hospital staff all moving through the busy main lobby in what looked like planned chaos. I wanted someone to blow a whistle and call for order.

Pale, disheveled patients in wheelchairs were being pushed outdoors for some fresh air. Visitors were bumping into one another trying to find the information desk. Doctors were hurrying to the cafeteria to grab a bite of lunch before...what? Slicing a brain or stomach open like they were carving into a steak?

I shuddered.

Norb and I found our way to the check-in area where Darlene and my brother John were waiting for us. Reassuring words, hugs, and kisses were exchanged, and we all took a seat in the crowded waiting room.

A family gathering. A life-threatening disease. There was a story unfolding here, and I wondered how it would end.

After a very nerve-wracking waiting period, we were called upstairs to, uh huh, another waiting room. Eventually, I was led into a small cubicle where I undressed, put on a hospital gown, and climbed onto a gurney, hoping that the ever-so-comforting warm blanket was on the way. It came! Then I was given some pre-surgery information to be sure I understood the procedure, asked if I had any questions (*God, no, I already knew too much*), given some papers to sign, and read my Miranda rights. (Not really.)

When preparations were complete, my daughter, Norb, and John were allowed in one at a time for a brief visit before a nurse announced that Dr. Donahue was ready and I was whisked away. The last thing I remember saying as the doors to the operating room swung open and I saw the team waiting inside was, "Okay, let's do this!

After winning four or five rounds of hide-and-seek with the sun, the game was growing tiresome, so I sought other adventures. Fortunately, my eyes flashed open and I could see that I was back on earth. A somewhat blurry face with fuzzy black stuff on the chin loomed over me. It seemed familiar but somehow scary, so I shut my eyes quickly and zoomed back to outer space. A voice softly called, "Nanny," so I decided to take another shot at earth, and I opened my eyes long enough to see that it was my grandson, Chase. Relieved, I managed to mumble "Chase... beard!" before falling back into a dream state.

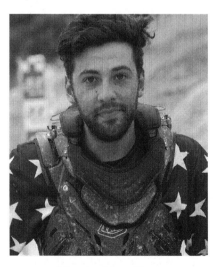

My grandson, Chase

CHAPTER 19

Spend All Your Kisses

I dozed on and off after my family left for the evening. Norb slept fully dressed on the guest couch in my hospital room. Located below the room's large picture window overlooking a portion of the UCLA campus, the couch was his bed for the next ten nights. I sat upright in my bed all night going through multiple stages of sleep. Every so often, I could hear the whirling blades of the emergency helicopter landing on the building next to the one I was in, but I had no interest in opening my eyes again. I let the humming sound lull me deeper into sleep.

When the pain worsened and woke me, I reluctantly pushed the button attached to my bed to release pain medication. I was afraid I might take too much, but medical staff told me it was controlled and "not to worry."

I suffered mixed emotions that first night after surgery. Dr. Donahue was pleased with the outcome of the operation. "It could not have gone better," he said when I awoke. "We checked ten or more of your lymph nodes and no sign of cancer." So why was I feeling so despondent now? Maybe it was the stress leading up to the operation, not knowing the outcome. Maybe realizing that I'd had a close brush with death was finally taking its toll. Maybe the drugs.

My thoughts drifted back to my grandson planting a kiss on my cheek earlier that day. He's a handsome twenty-four-year-old, over six feet tall, and he still calls me "Nanny." That kiss was comforting. I could feel my lips begin to curl into a smile as I recalled the time I did the same to my own beloved grandmother as she lay in a hospice bed many years ago.

Her name was Ann, but she was known to us as "Nana," what most Italian grandmothers were called by their grandchildren. When my first grandchild, Taylor, was born, we already had a "Nana" (my mother) and a "Great Nana" (my grandmother), so I opted for "Nanny." Close enough, I thought, and it would save us all from having to deal with yet a third living "Nana." (The five-generation photo we took a few months later was amazing!) *My* Nana was the matriarch of the family, and she never let us forget it was her *only* purpose in life.

Nana was born in the tiny village of Maddaloni, in the province of Caserta, Italy, where her father was the mayor of the town. The family arrived in America by boat when she was twelve and settled in what was then an Italian neighborhood near East 120th street and Pleasant Avenue in Manhattan. Like most Italian immigrants, her family worked in a clothing factory for many years, which allowed my grandmother to obtain an education and eventually, with hard work, lead a middle-income lifestyle.

Nana never wanted to return to Italy, although I offered to take her several times. "What do I want to go back to the old country for?" she'd snap, adding emphasis with a few Italian hand-waving gestures, as though there was something the matter with me for even *suggesting* such a thing. "Everything I want is right here," she'd insist. But she brought a lot of those old-country ideas with her. As she aged, she took her role of "Matriarch" even more seriously, much to the chagrin of her children and grandchildren. She had an endless stream of orders that she barked out at us all the time: "Cut your hair, get a job," to the boys, and my own personal favorite aimed at me was, "Eat something, for crying out loud. You're skinny as a stick."

On many Sunday mornings—growing up in the Bronx, where the family eventually relocated—I'd stop by Nana's on my way "to church." Of course, I knew she would insist on making me a bowl of oatmeal and a cup of hot cocoa. Soon after, fortified against the cold New York winter, I'd make my way up Southern Boulevard as I fingered the few coins Nana had shoved in my pocket for the collection box. I can still picture her leaning out of the sixth-story window—neck outstretched so she could see beyond the bars of the fire escape—to be sure I was headed in the direction of St. Athanasius. I'd smile and wave and, more often than not, when I was safely out of sight, turn left and head around the block to work my way back to our apartment on Fox Street. But not before stopping at a local candy store where I gave a silent sign of the cross before exchanging those coins for something much more soul-lifting than any sermon an eight-year-old could imagine—a chocolate egg cream.

As children, we foolishly tried to argue back to Nana, and as adults we merely tolerated her meddlesome ways, but I'm not sure we really understood how much she loved and wanted to protect us. I often tried to get her to talk about her past, but in her mind, it was a waste of time. I marveled that she was born before the Wright brothers took their first flight in 1903. "Imagine that!" she said matter-of-factly when I mentioned it to her one day.

I wondered if I had underestimated the richness of her experiences as she saw one development after another change the world around her: the telephone, the automobile, television, washing machines. And that these "luxuries" made us less dependent on her and her old-fashioned ways, and were a threat to her role as head of the family. "Family is everything," she'd always insisted. "Keep the family together," was one of the last "orders" she gave as she lay weakened and close to death on my last visit with her.

She was asleep when I entered her room on a snowy afternoon in upstate New York in the late '90s. I leaned over and kissed her cheek. Her pale skin felt as soft as rose petals. She didn't stir. I moved over to the chair near a window on the opposite side of the room and caught the last glimpse of evening light as it glistened across the expansive, snow-covered lawn below the hill where the hospice was perched. Jetlagged from the flight to New York, the train trip upstate and the car ride to the hospital, my eyes grew heavy and I fought sleep. Minutes later, I heard Nana moan softly, "More." Quickly moving back to the bed, I leaned over and whispered in her ear, "More what, Nana?"

"Kisses," she replied, her eyes still closed.

———— * * * ————

Several years after my grandmother passed away, I read a book called *Spend All Your Kisses, Mr. Smith*, which reminded me of my last visit with Nana. The book was written by a friend and colleague, Jack Smith, a witty columnist for the *L.A. Times*.

Jack's son was going to be married in Paris where his fiancé was from, but Jack did not want to go to France for the wedding. "I don't speak French, they eat little birds, and someone has to feed the cats," he argued. So, his wife, Denny, went alone. He agonized over his decision for a week before receiving a letter from her, which read in part: *It's not too late to change your mind. Spend all your kisses, Mr. Smith.*

It was a sentence he had read to her from a book of Greek or Roman poetry a year earlier, a sentence that he considered "remarkably good advice." "Surely," Jack wrote later in his book, "it meant there is no point in taking any of one's riches into the next world. Why keep a kiss, a gesture, a word that might give a moment's pleasure to someone else?" That night Jack booked a flight to Paris, and some months later, when I visited the Smiths, I noticed the words "Spend All Your Kisses" in a frame over his desk...and it warmed my heart.

Nana's "kisses" were steaming bowls of oatmeal on cold winter mornings and loose coins pressed into a child's mittens. She undoubtedly suspected those coins would end up on the counter of some corner candy store a few minutes later. In the end, she made a simple last request that cost me nothing and that I eagerly provided. I would have smothered her with kisses the whole night if I thought it would have kept her from dying.

Pain jolted my thoughts, and I again pressed the button that would quickly bring relief. As the drug began to work its' magic and I drifted off to sleep, I whispered, "More" into the silent, night-filled room and thought of all the kisses I have yet to spend.

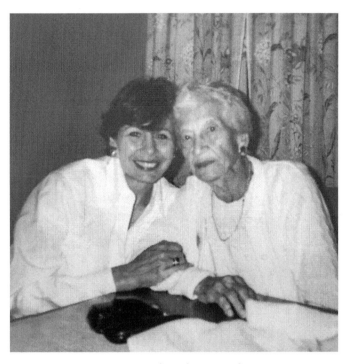

Nana-Our last photo together

CHAPTER 20

The Bald Spots

Both of my brothers visited me the next day. Frank is six years younger than I am, but he was stricken with lymphoma more than fifteen years ago. His regimen of extensive chemo and radiation was so debilitating we were sure we were going to lose him. I still recall the way he looked after one hospital visit that had me convinced it would be the last time I would see him. He'd lost all his teeth, his tongue was swollen, his skin was falling off, and he was almost skeletal from all the weight he'd lost.

But Frank survived it all. I remember thinking at the time how much I admired his courage and strength and wondered if I could have been as brave, had it been me. Now I'm being given that same chance.

My brother John is twelve years my junior (I still secretly think of him as "my baby brother" but have never said that to him). He's had his own bout with cancer—prostate—and also, thankfully, survived.

Frank is living with neuropathy and other lasting side effects of the treatment, but his spirits are high and he can often be seen riding around Grants Pass—the Oregon town where he lives—on his Harley Davidson.

John, when not working, divides his time between sailing his boat to Catalina and riding around on his Harley. I am encouraged by the fact that cancer has not prevented either of them from pursuing the active lifestyle they enjoyed before their illnesses. They give me hope that I can soon resume my active lifestyle—dancing, lifting weights, and the really challenging stuff—tossing salads, flipping pancakes, and twirling pizza dough in my kitchen.

Both of my brothers have been losing their hair for years and are now totally bald. We could not resist the temptation to put our heads together, so to speak, for this hilarious photo I call "The Bald Spots."

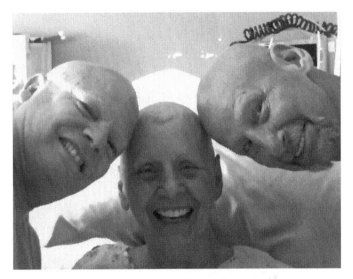

With brothers, John and Frank

CHAPTER 21

False Alarm!

The days passed and each day got better. On day three, I was able to eat and could order pretty much anything on the menu at any time of day—a neat idea I wished all hospitals would adopt. Day six came...and went. When my blood pressure soared to 190 over whatever, the anticipated six days turned into ten.

My hospital room was private, large, comfortable, and filled with state-of-the-art equipment. A huge picture window looked out onto a soccer green, and I could see the helicopter landing day and night one building over. I wondered if they were bringing in injured or ill patients, or doctors to handle emergency situations. Probably both.

Darlene and Taylor visited one day and brought Versailles restaurant's slow-simmered pork-and-cilantro rice for our lunch. In case you haven't figured it out by now, the three of us are "foodies!" When they were growing up, I got tired of preparing ordinary meat-and-potato meals every day, so I decided to expand my repertoire and took a gourmet cooking course from Rita Leinwand, the first woman to graduate from Cordon Bleu. The recipes were so delicious that I bought her cookbook, *How to Beat Those Cordon Bleus*. That started me on a quest to be more creative in my search for exquisite tastes, using unique ingredients and attempting more challenging techniques. Both of the girls followed me down that path and are excellent cooks. So, of course they had to bring food from one of their favorite restaurants. They knew how to cheer me up.

After we finished lunch, the girls decided to walk around the hallway to stretch their legs. I think it was the only time I broke down and cried in the hospital, despite all the pain and discomfort; I wanted to go with them! But I was still tethered to an IV pole, oxygen, drainage tubes, and leg boots. I suddenly wondered if I'd ever be able to walk with them again, and my heart sank. They were concerned when they returned and found I'd been crying, but just seeing their faces brought me joy and reminded me how lucky I was to be alive and have such a loving family. On their next visit, I was able to walk with them. It was slow going, and I pushed an IV pole all the way to a sunny patio with one hand while holding my gown closed with the other. But I was out walking with my girls, so things were looking up.

One evening a few days later, I was feeling dizzy, as though I was about to pass out. So, I pushed the "call" button and asked for a cold rag to put on my forehead. I have a history of fainting spells, and, if caught early enough, the coldness usually brings me out of them. Within seconds, the door was thrown open and a half-dozen nurses flew into the room. One of them was holding a fire extinguisher. She scanned the room and, finding nothing to be alarmed about, squinted her eyes at me as she would a naughty child.

"Did you call *code red*?" she asked in a scolding tone.

"No," I said meekly. "I just asked for a *cold rag*."

The room got quiet, and I could sense the nurses' frustration as they began filing out one by one. I started to utter, in my defense, that I didn't think patients were even *allowed* to call "code red," but that seemed a moot point now.

I never got the cold rag. They did offer me a sleeping pill though.

CHAPTER 22

Joy Is Not the Absence of Pain.

—Ayn Rand

The drive home from the hospital was more difficult than I had anticipated. Actually, it was friggin' miserable. Perhaps I should have gone down to Darlene's in Laguna as originally planned, but the extra time in the hospital made me anxious to get back home and into my own bed.

Norb opened the front door. I made a beeline for my bedroom, briefly noticing the softness of the new, mustard-colored carpet installed in my absence. *Thank you, Di. You pulled it off*! I staggered toward my bed.

The pain was worsening but so was my stubborn resistance to taking the Norco. I had been cutting the dosage in half, then quarters, because the drug made me feel out of control and Virgos hate that. We want to be in control most of the time. Okay, *all* the time. (We've been over this!)

So, I crawled into bed and hoped stillness would ease the pain. Norb went into the living room, leaving me to rest quietly. But the pain got so intense that I couldn't take it anymore, and I screamed at Norb, "Bring me the Norco, NOW!" He came running with the pills and a glass of water. By the time he reached me, I had curled up in a fetal position, clutching my stomach, crying hysterically, and cursing myself for letting the pain get ahead of me. Frightened beyond imagination, I begged Norb not to leave me. He immediately got under the covers, wrapped himself around my trembling body, and began to rock me gently.

"I won't leave you, baby. I'm right here. It's going to be all right."

"Don't leave me," I cried over and over in my worsening panic.

"Shhhh," he said as his grip tightened and he continued to rock me. "The meds will kick in soon. I'm right here, and I won't leave you."

As the Norco took effect, I could feel my body begin to relax, and I soon fell into a heavy sleep.

When I awoke, the pain was gone, and Norb, still beside me, dozed comfortably. I lay quietly, not moving, thankful that the pain had diminished so quickly. Thinking back on the past hour of excruciating pain, I was reminded of an Ayn Rand quote I had read many years ago in her novel *Atlas Shrugged*. In discussing emotions, Rand begins with the premise that "joy is not the absence of pain." I understood and accepted the concept immediately, but never was it more self-evident to me until now. To not feel pain, physical or emotional, is a good thing, but it is a neutral feeling at best. Joy comes when you awake to find yourself wrapped in the arms of someone you love.

CHAPTER 23

Frankenstein and Wine

It was time for the staples to come out. Jeannie drove me down to UCLA. We took Highway 1 instead of Interstate 5 so we could stop for breakfast at Well Bread in Los Alamos on the way down and San Ysidro Inn in Montecito for lunch on the way home the following day. I mean, we were going right by them both. And we had to eat, didn't we?

Frankenstein did NOT have to go through the removal of stitches, and if he had, I have no doubt he would have screamed bloody murder, pansy-ass monster that he was.

I did not scream. Though I was ready to. The thought of that staple remover attacking a still painful area of my tummy—snip, snip, snip, one at a time till all twenty staples were yanked out—had me terrified.

It almost kept me from enjoying that poached egg gently encircled by a slice of crusty country bread with shaved Romano cheese and roasted celebrity tomatoes at Well Bread.

But to be honest, it wasn't that bad (the stitch removal, that is...the breakfast was great!). Kudos again to UCLA. I decided I would bring the team a case of wine on my next trip down to L.A. Maybe some of my favorite blends from Guyomar or a selection of pinot noir from Windward. Actually, Guyomar would be more appropriate. They make fabulous wine, and the "pick-up" party they hosted that year had landed me in the hospital—thank goodness!

The evening of the fateful party was warm and pleasant. Tables were set up outside with a view of the grapevine-covered rolling hills in the background. The music was delightful and the wine and appetizers—cheese, bread, olives, and selected meats—were delicious. Many in my Wine Diva group were also present. When dinner was announced, I was awed by the extent of the buffet table containing barbecued pork, beef, chicken, lamb and shrimp, along with an abundance of rice, beans, salads, and more. Yeah, I sampled it all!

For months prior to that evening, I had been experiencing pain under the left breast, but several tests had failed to find a cause. That night, after the party, the pain worsened and lasted on and off for ten days. When I called Dr. Meiselman, he suggested a more invasive test, which, fortunately, exposed the tumor. If I hadn't been such a glutton, uh, been tempted by that deliciously prepared feast to consume much more than I usually do—the tumor might have gone undetected for months or longer, perhaps moving from stage two to three or four and ultimately rendering it inoperable.

So, you see why I had to marry the winery that helped save my life with the hospital staff that did save my life?

Not that I was drinking a lot of wine at the time; wine was on one of the "don'ts" during chemo, and I missed it, as I did my Wine Diva group. We had been making an impressive attempt to try all three hundred or so wineries in the area when we first formed ten years ago, visiting three wineries on the first Tuesday of every month. After five or so years, we cut it down to two wineries each time, but now we can only manage one tasting along with a picnic lunch at the winery or a nearby restaurant. Wine ages well over time. Wine Divas...well, not so much.

CHAPTER 24

A Year of
Living Dangerously

As I write, 2016 is drawing to a close, and I reflect back on the changes that living with cancer has made in my life; well, not changes so much as clarity—seeing things in focus or from a different perspective. I realize now more than ever how fortunate I am to be alive and to be surrounded with such kindness, love, and support from friends in this wonderful community and from Norb and my family, who, despite the distance, spent more time with me than I could ever have hoped for.

In October, I was given the opportunity to play a leading role in *Love Letters* at the local Cambria Center for the Arts and Theatre. Though I was barely healed from the operation and would be starting chemo again soon, studying the script and attending rehearsals kept my mind focused on the future.

Although the role would be challenging, I felt I could do it. (Thank you, Nancy Green, for taking a chance on me.) My biggest concern...should I go au naturel (bald) or cover my head? I ultimately decided on a scarf. The vanity thing, again.

Darlene and Taylor drove up for the performance that weekend. Taylor even helped me with makeup. "I don't have any brows or lashes," I moaned as I gazed at my face in the mirror.

"Yes, you do. I just need to color them in more," she said, grabbing some sticks and wands. What an improvement she made, and I breathed a sigh of relief.

Darlene, Taylor, and I have a "girl's theatre night" and try to see a live show once every year, usually at the Pantages Theatre in Hollywood: *Fiddler on the Roof* a few years ago, *The Book of Mormon*, *Hamilton*, and, more recently, Andrea Bocelli at the Hollywood Bowl. Well, Cambria is not Hollywood, but it was "Nan" in a leading role and not to be missed, despite the five-hour drive. Norb came, too, and I was grateful for their never-ending support.

My sneaky daughter also threw a surprise birthday party for me back in August at a local winery. "Let's go to Oso Libre for the sliders," she said while visiting that weekend. I love their sliders, so I thought it was a great idea. Plus, it's a beautiful outdoor location in Paso Robles, about a thirty-five-minute drive from Cambria. When we arrived and headed toward the rear where the sliders are served, I was shocked to hear "surprise" shouted out by many of my Cambria friends. She had to have been planning it for months. I was overwhelmed

I spent Thanksgiving with the family in Laguna, and after dinner we played a card game I was not familiar with. We weren't in teams, but the game allowed a player to "target" another player and put that player at a disadvantage when it was his or her turn; the targeted person usually ended up being the one who was leading in points. Chase, at one point, targeted me, and I shamefully responded in the whiniest voice I could muster.

"How could you do this to me, Chase? Did you forget about (sniff, sniff) that whole cancer thing and..."

Needless to say, I won that game.

The family all drove up to Cambria for Christmas, and we attended a wonderful Holiday Bazaar at the local lodge. It took a million lights to create this fantasy walk through the woods with animated exhibits and fairytale scenes, craft booths, music, and, of course, lots of food and drink.

Later, we opened Christmas presents sitting near a tiny tree I had managed to decorate for the gathering. Darlene was the first to open a gift from Taylor—a microgreen kit. I'm not a big salad eater nor am I much of a gardener, so I said laughingly, "I'm glad I didn't get one of those." Their turn to laugh as guess what the next package for me to open contained?

Chase is planning a move to Colorado so I typed

this message and tucked it inside a Christmas card for him.

"In preparation for your trip to cold country, I'm sending you a gift certificate from REI. (Check your email now!) Merry Christmas. Love, Nan.

P.S. Can you show me how to find emojis on my computer? I wanted to include a Christmas tree or a heart but couldn't figure it out." Everyone roared when he read that last line, but I was serious. Note to self: *Sign up for classes at the Apple store in January.*

Norb was away that weekend, so I left his gifts to me unopened but did tear into the two cards he had sent me. The front of one card read, "Do you know why Santa comes down the chimney?" And on the inside: "Who knows why men do *anything?*" That went a long way in explaining how he could have chosen the second card, which read: "Fuck, yeah, I wish you a Merry Christmas!"

A week or so later, I spotted the microgreens under the tree and thought, *What the heck. Might as well give 'em a try.* So, I placed them in the sun, just like Taylor said. But when I checked a few days later... nothing!

Apparently, you're supposed to take them out of the box.

And water them.

CHAPTER 25

Two to Five

Two to five, I say.

Two to five what? you ask
Dollars you spend on a latte?
Times you exercise each week?
Books on your list to read?
Ways to say, "I love you?"

Two to five, I say.

Two to five what? you ask again
Cakes you have to bake?
Cups you have to wash?
Closets you have to clean?
Clocks you have to wind?

Two to five, I say

Two to five what? you shout impatiently!
Trees you'd like to plant?
Hills you'd like to climb?
Paths you'd like to walk?
Promises you'd like to keep?

Two to five, I say

Two to five what? you scream in exasperation!
Hours you have to wait for the cable guy?
Minutes you need to scramble an egg?
Seconds it takes a newborn to breathe?
Years of life expectancy after the Whipple?

The last one...I say.

CHAPTER 26

Dragon Slayer

I was checking the Pancreatic Cancer Action Network's website for some nutritional advice when I spotted an article on survival rates for those who had undergone the Whipple procedure, which, of course, included me. The chilling words "two to five years" stabbed me in the chest. I spent the entire day walking around the house repeating *two to five, two to five* over and over in my head until, hoping to clear my mind, I wrote the words down and then I went to bed.

By morning, my fighting spirit was back in control, and I asked myself, as I often had in the past when faced with daunting challenges, *how many dragons do I need to slay today?*

Just one, came the reply, *but it's a doozie!* Well, I was no stranger to doing battle.

——— ✻ ✻ ✻ ———

I was raised in the South Bronx—which itself is a testament to my survival skills—in a very strict Italian family (ditto!) in the early 1940s. My grandparents, a no-nonsense set of immigrants, preached hard work and self-reliance and asked for nothing except the opportunity to succeed and, oh yes, for God to bless their wonderful adopted country. Some of their stricter ideas from "the old country" (children should be seen and not heard; You made your bed, you lie in it; do as I say, not as I do) seemed harsh when I was a child.

My grandfathers were sweet and gentle souls, but my grandmothers ruled with an iron fist. They would have sent chills down the spines of Joe Bananas, Frankie Fingers, and Ice Pick Willie. They were tough on us kids but for good reason. They loved us and thought America would spoil us. How could we grow up strong and self-reliant in this land of so much freedom and wealth? But I grew to respect their strength and determination, which they practiced against great odds, to carve out a better life for themselves and their families.

My father must have recognized my fighting spirit early on. Inspired by a photo of me at about a year old—bundled up in a snow outfit, standing stiff-legged, fists clenched, and a scowl on my face that warned I was ready to do battle, if only against the cold—he nicknamed me "Butch." "You look like a little toughie," he'd tease and lightly knuckle me on the chin. Dad had the name embossed on a tiny medal of St. Christopher he gave me when I was eleven and Mom, now re-married, had decided to move us to California. "To watch over you," he said with tears in his eyes, not knowing when he'd ever see me again.

As a scrawny and unkempt teenager attending a California junior high school in the last year, when all the clicks had already been formed, I felt—no, was—an outsider. But it was worse than that. In New York, the junior high schools were separated by gender: the boys went to one public school and the girls to another. (The schools at the time were numbered, PS 60 or PS 62.) Here in my new school, named after Benjamin Franklin, it seemed unnatural and awkward at my age to be thrust in with boys so suddenly. My New York accent didn't help either. "Say Waudah," or "chalk-lit," the kids would tease. I worked hard that year to get rid of my accent so I wouldn't stand out as much. And since my mom didn't allow me to participate in afterschool activities because I had to get home and watch my two younger brothers, do chores, and make dinner, the opportunity to find friendship in sports or other after-school clubs was not possible. I was friendless and lonely, but in spite of it all, I liked learning and studied hard.

In high school, I joined a drama class, and, from that point on, my life changed. Dramatically! On the first day, Mrs. Gillian instructed me to go on stage and improvise an ice cream cone! I was petrified. I racked my brain for a clue. Nothing! I began to sweat. Then, remembering the photo of "Butch" on that snowy day, I assumed the same frigid pose—scowl and all. To my surprise, everyone laughed, including Mrs. Gillian.

I learned that I could be anyone but me up on that stage, and that was fine; an "anyone" might be better at making friends. Three years later, in my senior year, I won the Best Actress of the Year award, partly for having written and produced a comedy casting only male class members—most of whom were on the football team—and myself in all the roles. (I wasn't stupid.) I knew I was risking the ire of the girls in the class—all that rehearsal time behind the curtain with the boys—but it was worth it.

Shortly after I won the award, Hollywood sent out a casting call to the local schools to "send us your best" for tryouts in the new movie "West Side Story." The studio originally wanted all unknowns in the leading roles, and high school drama classes were a good source of undiscovered and, undoubtedly, inexpensive talent.

That year's Best Actor winner and I were picked up outside the school in a limo and driven to the studio, where we were interviewed in separate rooms. To my disappointment, I wasn't given the chance to read for the part. I was told my blue eyes were the problem as "Puerto Ricans did not have blue eyes." I figured that meant I just wasn't pretty enough. Or maybe they were hoping for someone with a New York accent?

But they did treat us to lunch in the commissary

before the drive back to school, where we were welcomed as heroes, although neither of us got a role in the film. I was comforted later when seeing the movie that it took someone as beautiful and as talented as Natalie Wood to steal—er, win—the part away from me. To this day, it's still one of my favorite movies because it reminds me of the old neighborhood on Fox street where I grew up, and the loving family I left behind.

In my senior year, I became interested in the law and talked of going to college, but my mother kept telling me that "college is a waste of money for girls as they only went to find husbands." She may have had a point. It was the sixties, and we couldn't afford college anyway, so I did what I was programmed to do: marry and have children. A house with a white picket fence and kids running around did hold a lot of appeal for me, but the marriage failed, and before a divorce could be filed, I found myself a widow with three young children to care for. Well, I had made my own bed, and it was time to lie in it. I would have to become...my grandparents.

I took some college night courses when I could, studying history and philosophy—my favorite subjects. I was impressed with and influenced by many of the great thinkers and writers I discovered along the way: Aristotle and his reliance on reason and logic as guiding principles; Ayn Rand and her insistence that, as rational beings, we must trust the validity of our own minds; Thomas Jefferson and his insatiable appetite for knowledge; and Thomas Paine's as one of the first to fight for individual liberty and the rights of man. I was charmed by the wit of Mark Twain. I admired the wisdom of Winston Churchill, the courage of Galileo, the beauty and sensitivity of Rudyard Kipling's poems, and was awed by Hemingway's adventures. Others I enjoyed were De Tocqueville, Hugo, McCullough and—for his ability to have me roaring with laughter—Bill Bryson. Bryson's *Notes from a Small Island*, which I discovered while living in London, inspired me to want to write in the same humorous style of his that gave me such pleasure. These are many of the favorites who had a positive impact on me through the years.

I loved my studies, but life wasn't easy. Often, I held two jobs in order to provide for my young children. I wanted them to have all the things I didn't have growing up. I worked as a secretary during the day and waitressed nights while my children slept. I never considered welfare. It wasn't in my DNA. What would my grandparents think?

In 1970, I landed a job in classified advertising sales at the *Los Angeles Times*. There were sixty women working the phones for ads. Commissions added up, and the job provided substantial benefits a single mother could rely on. But the more lucrative outside display ad sales positions were available only to men. They were allowed company cars, the ability to travel, expense accounts, and much greater opportunity for promotion into management. Not so for the gals.

However, six years later, when the *Times* was forced by the National Organization for Women to confront the issue, to their credit, they changed their policy. I quickly applied for a display sales job and, having had to interview with twelve male managers in a conference room, I felt like I was on trial. But I passed muster and was soon assigned an outside territory. Things were looking up!

I eventually worked my way up to sales manager of the Sunday magazines *Home* and *TV Guide*. When I was named national and international advertising manager, I was thrilled to death since the travel to Southeast Asia was a terrific perk. Several years later, when the *Times* decided to open a business office in London, I wasted no time applying for the job. I had been a widow for the second time and my children were grown and gone. How could I pass up such a wonderful opportunity? I was thrilled to get the job and spent the next five years traveling most of Europe syndicating US editorial content to European publications. For instance (and in the interest of full disclosure, *I have met with Russians*), I negotiated with a publication in Moscow to produce the Russian version of the *Sports Illustrated* swimsuit issue. (It was soon discovered that there is no Russian word for "bikini," but that didn't stop them.)

We also carried more serious contributors, such as Henry Kissinger, Jesse Jackson, Paul Samuelson. Publications included *USA Today*, the *Wall Street*

Journal, *Popular Science*, and many others. I later added the Russian news agency, TASS, to the list. The constant travel, the language, and the cultural and political differences made it a difficult, and at times, dangerous job. But it turned out to be the most interesting and rewarding five years of my entire career.

Soon after I returned to the United States, I was promoted to president of a small Times-owned company called Newscom, a state-of-the-art news and photo delivery service, where I remained until, after thirty-four years with the *Times*, I retired and moved to Cambria.

The scowling face is gone, I still hate the cold, and no one ever called me Butch except Dad, but maybe, just maybe, he was right and I really am "a little toughie."

Now where did I leave that sword?

2

Other Calamities

CHAPTER 27

Me and Galileo

What would a brilliant fifteenth-century Italian scientist have in common with a twenty-first-century aging American female with a bad hip? Torture! That's what.

▶ **EMAIL UPDATE: JANUARY 6, 2017**

As you know, this dang right hip has been acting up for the last two years and it is getting worse. So, my orthopedic doctor, Daniel Woods, ordered a dye-injected MRI in December and Norb and I went for the results a few days ago. Dr. Woods said that, because of severe arthritis, all the cartilage in the socket are gone. "You're bone on bone, and the only way to solve the problem is to have a hip replacement."

Yikes! Another operation? I'm still getting chemo!!! My jaw dropped.

Books and charts came out, Norb pulled his chair closer and all I heard was a lot of blah, blah, blah from the doctor and "Titanium? Cool," from Norb. More blah, blah, blah...blah, blah between the two of them.

I was still in a state of shock so when the doc asked, "Any questions?" I went completely blah-less and shook my head from side to side. Now, of course, I have about a hundred questions.

But the doc promised to send me the book with the picture of the splayed operating table that Norb said "looks like a torture rack, heh, heh." I didn't find that observation particularly amusing, but he was right! It did remind me of the instrument used to intimidate the scientist/astronomer Galileo.

Galileo was eighty when he was threatened with "the rack" for his belief in the Copernican theory that the sun, not the earth, is the center of the universe. He eventually recanted (who could blame him?) and was spared the torture, but I apparently have to suck it up. Punishment probably for my belief, at times, that I am the center of the universe.

Not to feel left out of this new development, my oncologist, darling Dr. "D," said I will have to wait six weeks after chemo ends before I can have the operation. My final treatment, for this round, is mid-February, so that gives me until late March to have some fun before the big day on...the rack. With recovery, I should be back to dance on a full-scale basis by May, making it a full year since this whole thing started.

In the meantime, I plan to show up and do what I can when I can because the music and your smiling faces, dancing feet, and occasional outbursts of (off-key) song have and will continue to have a great deal to do with my speedy recovery.

A dear friend brought me a prepared meal a while back with a little miniature dish taped to the package that read, "Look for something beautiful each day." I've been doing so and today, my dancing friends, that would be you. Thank you for all your love and support.

CHAPTER 28

Slaying the Dragon Slayer

My cell phone rang early one morning in February. I was still groggy with sleep but reached for the phone anyway and whispered, "Hello."

"Maryann, where are you?" the voice on the other end of the line asked excitedly.

"I'm at my daughter's in Laguna Beach. Why?"

"Oh! Thank goodness," breathed my friend Raimund with a sigh of relief. "A car crashed into the French Bakery this morning, and Judy and I know you have coffee there every day."

"What?!" I asked in shock. "Was anyone hurt?"

It seems many of the friends I sit and chat with most mornings had come and gone except for dear little Ruth, who suffered severe ankle damage and was hospitalized. A few other customers were also hospitalized, but fortunately nothing life-threatening. I discovered later that a car ran a stop sign, rammed into another car in the parking lot, and both crashed thru the wall of the shop right into the space I normally occupy.

I don't want to appear paranoid, but I've survived pancreatic cancer and a potentially fatal car crash in the last year, so I'm wondering where the next strike might come from and how much longer my luck will hold out.

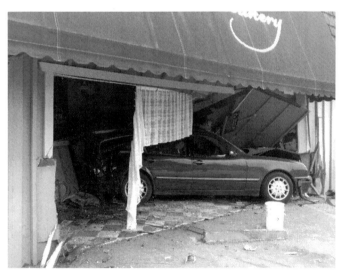

I'm not making this stuff up!

CHAPTER 29

Bionic Woman

Through the years, I've lost my tonsils, my appendix, a few annoying hemorrhoids, my entire uterus, my gall bladder, a parathyroid, part of my pancreas, my spleen, and my virginity without getting one damn thing in return. But this time, thanks to advanced medical science, I actually received a *replacement* part. A brand-spanking-new state-of-the-art hip made from titanium, plastic, ceramic, and metal. The operation was performed on a special table, the OI Hana, which boasts of having a robotic arm and almost guarantees you won't end up with one leg shorter than the other. I just hope it comes with a lifetime warranty. My lifetime, not the equipment's.

▶ **EMAIL UPDATE: MARCH 9, 2017**

Well, glad THAT's over!

Dr. Woods was very pleased with the outcome of the surgery. The follow-up game of "Find the Patient," not so much.

After recovery, I was brought to a room in the surgical unit. Because there was some overcrowding in that room, the supervising nurse decided to move me into another room to give me some needed post-surgery recovery time. But, there was no space available in the surgical unit so they sent me down to the intensive care unit for the night. Doctor Woods was sure surprised the next morning to find I'd gone missing. He found me but he wasn't amused.

They needed the ICU room back the next day and the only open bed was in the cardiac unit so I was moved there. The nurses had that, "Oh, just an ortho-patient, nothing much to see here," look on their faces so I passed out a few times to get their attention and to give them an opportunity to practice their heart monitoring-skills. I'm thoughtful that way.

The doctor found me again but I could tell he was running out of patience. Norb suggested he plant a GPS system in me so I would be easier to find, but the suggestion wasn't well received. Then a bed opened up in the surgical unit and I was moved yet again.

Finally, and I can't prove this, I think the Russians leaked my location because Dr. Woods showed up and signed my release papers on day three. Well, he didn't get rid of—er—release me so much as sign me over to the hospital staff doctor to find out why I was passing out. I never saw him on day four so his strategy appeared to have worked.

A few tests the next day failed to show anything amiss with my heart; at least not anything traceable after that handsome, young, staff doctor told me he was taking over my care. (sigh.) Anyway, turns out I'm sensitive to pain meds. (Yeah, I know that!)

But on the bright side, my therapist had quite a sense of humor. He had been working with me when I passed out twice in quick succession a day earlier. I told him later that I honestly didn't remember a thing. He smiled and said, "When you woke the first time, you told me I was the handsomest man you'd ever seen, and the second time…you borrowed fifty bucks!"

Don't even ask me about the third time. Okay, it was right after I saw what was on the lunch tray. Good thing Norb was there and willing to run out for decent provisions. Hospital food sucks!

As if this wasn't enough, I was later told by my sister-in-law, who is a surgical nurse, that the procedure is performed on the body naked from the waist down! What?

"Well, they have to be sure the hips and legs are all lined up evenly," she added with a subtle chuckle.

I suppose so, but did she have to leave me with that humiliating vision etched in my brain for the rest of my life?

P.S. An artist friend of mine drew a really "hip" card signed by all the girls in my aerobics class. It reads: "No Bones About It, you are super hip with us." I posted a picture of me (fully covered) holding up the card in room 306, or was it the ICU or the cardio unit or...?

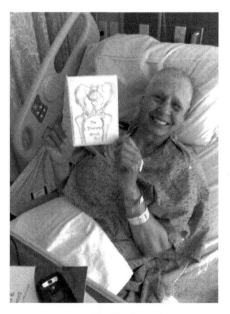

A really "hip" card

CHAPTER 30

I'm Alive,
So Why Not Shop?

► EMAIL UPDATE: APRIL 20, 2017

Went into town today to pick up a few things at Williams Sonoma. Arrived home with a pasta machine, a pizza oven, a torch for making crème brûlée, an infrared grill, a pressure cooker, some braising sauces, and a 2017 Mercedes Benz GLA 250 Crossover in a creamy-white with all the extras from Alfano Motors.

I was a little worried on the drive home that, since I hadn't even had my three-month post chemo checkup yet, spending all that money was probably a bit premature. Hmmm.

I might have to re-think that pasta machine.

CHAPTER 31

It's My Body and
I'll Cry if I Want to...

3 a.m. and my eyes pop open. Damn! I begin to toss and turn, hoping a change of position will lull me back to sleep. Often this works. Not tonight. I push hard on key muscles to get them to stretch and relax. In the dark, under the blankets, in some spots, it feels like me, but I'm not fooled. I want to love this body again, but in the morning, in the light, in the mirror, I will see all of those ugly scars.

The one high on my neck where the para-thyroid was removed, the puckered one on my chest where the port was inserted, the gall bladder scar, and the one shaped like a boomerang made by the removal of a good chunk of my pancreas and which now feels like a row of tiny cream puffs billowing out from under my left breast. And not to be ignored is the loaf of rye *rising* (forgive the pun) in the form of dense scar tissue on my right thigh where the hip was replaced.

Battle scars? Nothing so noble as that.

My head is bloody but not bowed, I'm reminded by Kipling.

So, I brush away the tears of self-pity and take pride in knowing I've survived it all. I'm not seventeen! That body no longer exists, but the soul is still intact, I think.

I rub my mid-section again where I can feel a huge eclair-shaped roll of scar tissue making itself at home. It occurs to me that it's also a place where, once upon a time, three adorable babies also made their home—temporarily. Well, then. Maybe I should cut it some slack.

3:15 a.m. I give up trying to sleep, turn on the light, and grab the book *Healthy Eating for Cancer Survivors* from the shelf near my bed. I turn to the chapter titled *Cancer Loves Sugar.* Humph! At least we have that much in common. I suppose I should eliminate sugar from my diet. But after seventy-odd years of eating sweets, I wonder, *If I gave it up now, how much more breathing time would it get me here on earth? An extra hour? A whole day? Maybe a week? Is the trade-off worth it?*

I toss the book back on the shelf. It lands on top of *The Joy of Chocolate* and *A Hundred Pizzas from One Easy Recipe.* I stretch out in bed, rub the sticky-pudding ridges on my tummy again and look at the clock. 3:39 a.m. Might as well check my email since I'm awake.

I'm back, and you won't believe this!

A message from my daughter, Darlene, sent at 11:30 p.m. the previous evening. The subject is "Yorkshire Pudding," and below the subject is a photo of two giant, puffed-up puddings (resembling fairly closely, the current condition of my stomach) under which she wrote:

"OMG, I found these, and they took me right back to your prime rib and Yorkshire pudding dinners every Christmas. Thanks for opening my eyes to incredible eats."

Well, if that doesn't take the cake! Proof that the foods we love are sometimes more about fondue—uh—fond memories than anything else.

4:15 a.m. I yawn, turn off the light, and snuggle under my warming blanket. Only three more hours and I can polish off the last one of those maple-pecan muffins I baked yesterday.

I'm not convinced I still love this body, but I know one thing for sure: the way I indulge its craving for sweets...this body still loves me!

CHAPTER 32

Ducking Bullets

I didn't survive pancreatic cancer only to be killed by a falling tree. After a heavy rain and the mudslides that usually follow here in the heavily forested area of Cambria, lots of trees have come down on Burton Drive where I curve my way around every morning on the way to the French Bakery. Well, no, it hasn't happened yet, but the way things are going, I wouldn't be surprised. First came the cancer threat and the Fishnet Stockings panic, followed by the asbestos scare, the torture rack, the lost-patient caper, the French Bakery incident, and the flaming infrared grill I had to return to Williams Sonoma because the bloody thing almost set my kitchen cabinets on fire. And today, a head-on collision on Highway 1 in my brand-new car. Not my fault! I was minding my own business at a red light when a car coming from the opposite direction ran the light and crashed into another car, pushing that car into the space that I was occupying. (Sound familiar?)

What next? Attacked by a mountain lion? Not impossible as there are many deer in the area, and mountain lions have been spotted roaming around the town. The advice if you see one is to not run. "Stand tall, wave your arms, and make a lot of noise," they say. Does screaming, "*What the fuck!!!*" at the top of your lungs count as noise?

Here's what's wrong with that plan. Since I was a child, I have had periodic fainting spells. "Petit mal," the doctors call them, but they can't explain why they happen. I can. It's when I'm scared stiff! A second-grade teacher calls me up to her desk to scold me, and down I go. I'm caught at the candy store with money meant for the collection box...down! Turbulence in the air, down! Earthquake, down! Out of wine! Uh...

So, back to the mountain lion, I think you can see where I'm going with this.

On the other hand, what fun would it be for the lion to have his prey simply crumble at his feet without a chase? A noble lion might poke me with his paw, nudge me with his nose or let out a slow, growling sound. Anything to get me up and running and give me a sporting chance. He has, I'm sure, a reputation to protect.

All of the above happened in one year, more or less. I don't believe in conspiracy theories, but my name must be on a list somewhere up there, and there's serious disagreement about whether my time is up or not. I'm considering a call to the FBI to let them in on some made-up crime stuff. I can use my Italian maiden name for credibility and I *was* born in New York, so there's that! Maybe they'll put me in the Witness Protection Program with a new identity. It might buy me a few more years until the "holder of the list" finds me. I'm catching on to this game now.

Did I just hear a lion roar?

CHAPTER 33

Fear Is a Reaction. Courage Is a Decision.

—Winston Churchill

Just a little more than a year after the operation, and I sometimes think, *my cancer may be back*. The thought hits me hard. Not the cancer itself—the revelation that I used the word *my*. The acceptance of it, the familiarity with it, the ownership of that dreaded disease by referring to it as "my cancer."

Don't we hold things that belong to us as good, desirable, worthy, or even cherished? Does the word "my" presuppose that the things that belong to us are good for us; things like my home, my career, my garden, my child, my love? Shouldn't cancer belong in the category used to describe words that distance themselves from us, like "that thief, that scoundrel, that crummy movie, that poison, that killer disease?"

Maybe it's just me, but I've decided I will never think of that horrible disease as *mine* again. So, let me start over.

I think the cancer may be back. I feel that gnawing little pain under the left breast that was ultimately diagnosed as a "tumor in the pancreas" according to Dr. Nice Old Man. (Notice he called it "the" pancreas, not "your" pancreas. I think I'm on to something with this theory.) I tell myself it's just residual pain from the operation, although that was almost a year ago. Maybe—and I'm leaning toward this explanation for obvious reasons—I strained myself lifting weights?

Should I be planting spring bulbs? Or updating my estate plan?

"Don't look back," I say when it occurs. There's much to be done if time is running out, and since I have no say in the matter—that's evidently up to the Creator or Nature or some power beyond my control—how does one go on? Winston Churchill, when asked by his wife how he withstood the constant barrage of attacks from Parliament after he almost single-handedly saved Western civilization, replied, "I just keep buggering on!"

Well, me too, Winnie. Me too!

But then, a few days later during a three-month checkup, Dr. DiCarlo told me my tumor marker was up. Not a great worry, but it should be trending down since the tumor was removed. Right? This, combined with the pain I've been having caused him some concern, so he ordered another CT scan even though I'd had one barely two months ago. As I was leaving his office, Taylor called my cell, and hearing her voice choked me up. I fought tears but was able to remain calm while we chatted. After the call, I let loose.

It wasn't helpful that the long drive home along the coast was during the largest rain storm of the season. The sky, the wind, the surf, and my emotions were all flustered and in turmoil. Talk about a perfect storm.

At home that night, I sat staring into space, trying to sum up the courage to behave normally: make dinner, check email, vacuum—anything to keep from crumbling to the floor like a puppet whose strings had just been cut. *Fear is a reaction,* I reminded myself. Then I took a deep breath and repeated over and over to myself, courage, courage, courage!

Okay, I sighed with all the resolve I could muster. *Starting tomorrow.*

CHAPTER 34

Speaking of Heaven

Well, I hadn't been, but work with me here. Assuming there is a heaven, and assuming I make it through, there must be some really cool benefits up there. For instance, I will never again have to hear myself ask, "Where the hell are my car keys?" or "How do I get this friggin' remote to work?"

It would be great if I could stop stressing over whether the food I eat is "sustainably grown" or if my yogurt is made from cows *not* treated with rBST or rBGH, although in really small type (I had to use a magnifying glass to see it) the label reads "*no significant difference between milk made from cows treated with rBST or rBGH and those not treated with rBST or rBGH!" Does this annoy anyone? *Anyone*??

The good news is, my book will be gluten-free, although it might be printed in a plant that may have been across the street from a company that used to make the labels that are stamped on gluten-free products...like Jello? Now, the place has been turned into a "safe-space" with cuddly dogs and counselors and coloring books, so not to worry.

I'm also obsessing over whether my clothes and sheets and dust cloths and hats and carpets are made from "organic fiber." I don't think marketing people should be let through those pearly gates lest they feel compelled to place their stamp of approval on my wings, which are made of...? Hmmm.

Are there schedules up there? I have to admit that sometimes—okay, pretty much always—I can be a bit annoying to others because I am a fanatic about showing up everywhere on time. I'm hoping for forgiveness on this issue. If I am twenty minutes early for an appointment, I consider myself ten minutes late. Not a problem on my own, but if I am waiting for others to get going, I start pacing the floor, checking my watch, opening and shutting the front door and then the squeaky garage door. I'll admit this can be annoying. I've even been known to start the car while others are just getting out of the shower.

"Patience is a virtue," I've been told repeatedly. But I'm with the guy who said, "Why does patience have to be a virtue? Why can't 'hurry the fuck up' be a virtue?" It wasn't me. Honest! And if I ever find out who first came up with this brilliant idea, I'd love to get together sometime for a hug. Preferably twenty minutes earlier than scheduled, because time is suddenly more precious than it ever was. That doesn't mean I want to be early for my own demise. I just don't want to be late.

Ever!

CHAPTER 35

Bucket List?

Maybe because I turn seventy-four this month or the realization that the cancer could return at any time, I've whipped myself into a frenzy of activity. I can't say no to anything. Some might feel differently if they thought their time was limited, and do just the opposite—more yoga, deep contemplation, gardening, quiet walks on the beach. Hell, no, not for me.

Everything I've been through this past year reminds me of another brilliant Churchill quote: "Nothing is so exhilarating than being shot at without result!" Yeah, that explains it! That's why I feel so enlivened with the energy to do, well, everything and *all at the same time.*

After much urging from friends who were receiving my e-mail updates, I took up the challenge and decided to write this book. I also resumed leading my aerobics and weight training sessions three times a week. I rejoined the local "flash-mob" group and committed to learning two new dances for our annual street performances. I auditioned for the play *Red Herring* and was offered a role in it, which I quickly accepted. I was asked to give a talk to our local Lions Club on my career in the syndication business for the *L.A. Times* and said, "Happy to do it." I joined a local writing group, The Rough Writers, who are helping me with the book. I was asked to be a model in a local fashion show, and, of course, I couldn't turn *that* down.

I've become maniacal about cooking all my old favorite recipes, nearly driving Williams Sonoma crazy special-ordering equipment, sauces, signing up for classes in pasta, pizza, and pie making, and guess what? All of this to happen in the same month! Did I mention I'm writing a book?

And then it came. A letter from the Neptune Society. Uncanny how they know!

"Time Stands Still for No One," read the headline. "Before you know it, a year has passed, then two. You start thinking about all those things you should do, but haven't," it went on. Of course, they were thinking along different lines. You know, ashes to ashes, dust to dust, that sort of thing. Not one to shy away from sensitive subject matter, they launched into a sales pitch on cremation as the "sensible choice." Their reasoning: "It's dignified, inexpensive, and has," wait for it, "less impact on our environment." Of course, what impact my decaying body would have on the environment was, say, number gazillion on my list of worries at the moment.

But they had a point about getting things done, so the idea that perhaps I should be making a bucket list entered my mind. Then I thought, *Well, I'm already doing all the things I want to do* (see above paragraph). On the other hand, there are a lot of things that get in the way and slow me down. Annoying things, time-consuming things, socially responsible and politically correct things that frankly just drive me nuts, and I don't feel I should have to do them anymore.

So instead of a bucket list, why not a "Fuck-it" list? For instance:

- Worry about my weight? *Fuck it!*
- Cover the gray in my hair? *Fuck that, too!*
- Consume more green drinks? *Not gonna happen.*
- Text with Millennials? *Nope!*
- Fasten my seatbelt? Drive the speed limit? *Fuck it! Fuck it!*
- Pay my taxes? *Fuck the IRS!*

Okay, maybe not that last one, but it's a good start, don't you think? And as for the Neptune Society, well, you know...

CHAPTER 36

A Dream

It's two o'clock in the morning. I lay *A Gentleman in Moscow,* a book I'm reading for the second time, on my bedside table and switch off the light. But I'm restless and sleep doesn't come.

I think about Count Rostov, who, having had the poor judgment to be born into a family of wealth and privilege, is under house arrest at the Metropole hotel in Moscow shortly after the Russian Revolution. The hotel is where Rasputin entertained the Czarina Alexandria and her court before he was brutally murdered. I stayed at the Metropole when I visited Moscow on business in the '90s. I can still envision the long, drab hallways where a sturdy, Russian, babushka-clad woman was stationed at an empty desk all hours of the day and night to keep watch on the goings on. She never spoke. She never moved. She just watched. The rooms were sparse, and food in the restaurant all came out of cans, I was certain. In *A Gentleman in Moscow,* the author, Amor Towles, promised a closer look at the hotel's history and I was anxious to read more about it.

When I left the Count, he was on the parapet of a roof of the six-story building where, it appeared, he was about to leap to his death. I've grown fond of the Count. He's witty and charming and courageous; he's made the best of his circumstances, including the loss of his family, his country estate, and all his belongings to the Bolsheviks. He's been reduced to living in a 120-square-foot room in the upper levels of the hotel, not far from where many of the hotel's staff reside. But he begins to lose hope that his country will survive the Revolution and...damn! I have fallen in love with Count Rostov, and I really don't want him to die!

My anger subsides, and I've drifted into a fitful sleep. Soon after, I hear an inner voice ask:

"What's troubling you?"

"I think I may be dying," I cry out.

"Perhaps...are you still okay with that?" the voice pressures me.

"Yes, no...maybe," I cry.

"The last time we had this heart-to-heart you were prepared to..."

"I know, but that was before..."

"Before what?"

"Before I realized I was invincible."

"What? When did you become invincible?"

"When I beat the odds of surviving pancreatic cancer...and some other stuff. Have you not been paying attention? Four operations in as many years? I was beginning to think..."

"Well, if you're invincible, then how could you be dying?" the voice asks dismissively.

"You're just trying to confuse me."

"But when you were first diagnosed, you said..."

"I know what I said. But the- truth is, we really don't want to die!"

"We?"

"The Count and I."

"Well, that's easy. Just don't turn any more pages."

The heater's thermostat clicks on, and the sound snaps me back to reality. I defy my subconscious, reach for the book, and turn to the next page. Count Rostov moves closer to the parapet, then suddenly hears a familiar voice call his name. Perhaps an issue has arisen in the dining room and his help is needed. I wonder, *can they not locate the Chateauneuf de Pape? Mon Dieu!*

The voice urges him down from the parapet. I let out a deep sigh of relief as I lay the book, once again, on the table and switch off the light. I pull the blankets up over my head, snuggle into the softness of my pillow, and take comfort in knowing that Count Alexander Ilyich Rostov will not die tonight.

And neither will I.

CHAPTER 37

I've Been Through Hell and I'm Not Gonna Take It Anymore!

I suppose I'm not alone, but after a battle with cancer, a survivor might feel a bit, well, self-indulgent. This petulant attitude manifested itself in small ways that were important to no one but me. For instance:

A few years ago, I bought a creamy-white electric blanket for my bed. I've never appreciated it as much as I do now that all the treatment is over. I turn it on an hour or so before retiring, and the sheets are warm and comforting when I slip under the covers. I smile to myself, flutter my arms and legs in snow-angel fashion, and snuggle up for a heavenly night's sleep. But a few weeks ago, it stopped working. DRAT! I originally purchased it on line, so the next morning I contacted the manufacturer, who, since I was within the guarantee period, offered to send me a new one.

I could hardly wait for it to arrive, and when it did, I tore open the package and pulled it out of its protective plastic bag, but, "Gasp!"—it wasn't white! It was beige, and reminded me of what sink water looks like after you rinse off mushrooms or cow dung or...

I can't sleep under a beige blanket! Not when everything else on the bed is white! After what I've been through lately, I should be able to know at the end of the day, that all is well in this room—my sanctuary—under my lovely matched bedding. Life is good: no chemo here; no hospital, oncology center, or nausea; and no off-color blankets that disturb my equilibrium. But I was beginning to feel like a whiney baby, so I made the bed up and put it on anyway, even though everything else on my bed was white! Sheets! Comforter! Spread! Shams!

"Not so bad," I said to myself as I crawled into bed. I hid the blanket under the comforter so I couldn't see it, but I knew it was there. And that made it impossible to sleep.

I have always liked white, but lately, for some reason, it's become my favorite thing. I thought about "whiteness" every night when I got into bed. It was... clean, pure, healthy-looking, an uncompromising absolute: snug-able, and wrap-able. Beige, not so much. Beige can't make up its mind what it wants to be. It screams, "I can fit in anywhere!"

"NO!" I argued. "Not here, not ever!" So, I tore it off the bed and called the manufacturer the very next morning to tell them I wanted to exchange this ugly imposter for the real thing in white.

"Sorry, we're all out of the white, you'll have to keep the beige," the gal muttered unsympathetically into the phone.

Oh yeah? It took about five seconds to pull Amazon up and search for a white electric blanket. Of course, they had one *by the same manufacturer,* so I hit the "Buy now with 1-click" button, and it was on its way. If you've been through cancer, you seek comfort wherever you can find it.

I sent the beige one to Taylor, who was thrilled to have it, even though she hid it under *her* white comforter.

Ah, youth!

CHAPTER 38

Should I Kill Myself or Have a Cup of Coffee?

—Albert Camus

What was I thinking? I'd like to get every one of those who encouraged me to write a book and wring their necks. They told me so often, "Your updates are so funny, so inspiring, so entertaining, you should write a book!" that I decided to do it. Easy for them to say. They're not the ones lying awake night after night trying to think of how to end the bloody thing. It was Hemingway (or maybe a guy named Smith) who said, "Writing is easy...all you have to do is sit down at a typewriter and bleed." I've bled buckets, but I'm *still* not finished. (And neither is the book!)

Maybe I need another catastrophe to inspire me. Maybe I'm best under pressure. Maybe if that tree had fallen on me, I'd be able to come up with something, anything, to finish it off. Or finish me off. Where do I go from here? Should I be working on an Epilogue or an Epitaph? I could hug a tree the next time lightning strikes. *There's* a final chapter! Only, who would write it?

But for now, I want to get on with life! I've family to visit. I've pizzas to make. Pies to bake. Dances to choreograph. And weeds to feed—er—pull. I'm not getting any younger. The book has to end NOW!

Desperate for an idea, I sought inspiration from other authors and wondered how, say, Hemingway might end it. Hmmm!

I think that it is finished. But sometimes I think that it is not finished. Sometimes I cannot think. As I clutch the final pages to my chest, I tell myself there are enough words, or not enough words, but if there were more, it would be less, and the world would destroy it and me along with it because it's cruel that way, and I feel the bitterness as I stand here in the dark of night. Alone. In the rain.

Of course, there's always Option B. If I stall long enough, the unfinished book may outlive me, and maybe that idea of family and friends finishing it is not a bad one. Then it will be *their* problem.

The Epilogue would read: *I was concerned that I might not live long enough to fin...*

And the Epitaph would read: *I was right!*

CHAPTER 39

Spoiler Alert: I'm Still Here

During one of the first strength-training sessions after my return, I was leading the group in tri-cep overhead extensions.

"Right arm to left shoulder: one, two, three," I began.

One of the girls blurted out that she was really beginning to feel the effects of building muscle.

"I was carrying the vacuum up the steps and mentioned to my husband...."

"Four, five, six," I continued.

"...how much easier it was since I began weight training."

"Seven, eight, nine," I huffed.

"He was really proud of me," she added.

"That's your goal? Ten, eleven, twelve...," I asked in

astonishment... "to be a more efficient housekeeper?... thirteen, fourteen." Mine is to jog along the beach in a Baywatch swimsuit looking like I'm still twenty-one... twenty-two, twenty-three...and switch!"

I was joking, of course. One should not have unrealistic goals—like surviving pancreatic cancer. But then...

CHAPTER 40

R-E-S-P-E-C-T

In the last few weeks, every time I turn around, some-one is dying of pancreatic cancer. In a TV series I'd been watching, one character is a doctor who has just been diagnosed with cancer. He became distraught and withdrawn, refusing to undergo any treatment, despite the urging of his wife to do so.

"Why won't you talk to me about this," she pleads with him. "We need to have a treatment plan." Tired of her constant pressure, he shouts, "You don't under-stand. I've got pancreatic cancer. There is no cure. I am going to die!"

Well, shit! My head jerked away from the TV, but it was too late. The words had already penetrated my brain, and the immediate response was to fist-punch the couch pillow before reaching for the remote.

A few days earlier, I had been shopping at Marine Layer, my favorite little retail store in town for casual wear. The young salesgirl and I had become friendly, and she was aware of my bout with cancer. She always greeted me with a big smile and a hug when I walked in, as she did on that day, and asked me how I was feeling.

"I'm great," I answered. "I'm really doing well."

"Do you mind if I ask you what kind of cancer you had?" she asked with some hesitation.

"Pancreatic," I responded immediately.

"My mother is going through that now," she said with tears welling in her eyes.

I was shocked! Another salesgirl in the store overheard the conversation and walked over to us. She hadn't been aware. In a second, the three of us stood arms wrapped around each other in a circle of hugs and tears. I tried to assure her all would be well, but she had been led to believe there was very little hope. I cried for her. And I cried for me. Fear that the dreaded disease would come back to claim me, as it has so many others.

A week later, I overheard a friend mention that his sister-in-law had pancreatic cancer and that he and his wife had plans to meet with her the following day. He was distraught and appeared not to know what to expect, so I approached him and told him I'd been through it, and survived. I told him how the Whipple procedure saved me, and let him know that if he needed any more info, I'd be happy to help.

When he returned later that week, he told me there would be no operation, and that they had given the woman only six months to live. I couldn't help remembering that even survivors of the Whipple operation are given just two to five years life expectancy, and only nine percent make it past five years. I was approaching my second year in a few short weeks and had recently experienced some very familiar stomach pain. Real or imagined? I began to dread the approach of a CT scan scheduled for the following month.

When I switched on the news a few days later, Aretha Franklin's "R-E-S-P-E-C-T" was playing, and, as I knew she'd been ill, my first thought was that she probably had died. I am a great fan of Aretha's, having grown up with her music and loving it all. We even shared the same birth year—1942. "R-E-S-P-E-C-T" was one of the tunes I used for our aerobic workout sessions, and, as I was searching my files to find it so I could play it the following day, the words, "Aretha died after a losing battle with pancreatic cancer," rang from the TV anchor's lips. I almost hit the floor. I couldn't help feeling there was a strong warning in the stories of the last few weeks—a warning I've been trying to ignore.

I did play "R E S P E C T" in tribute to Aretha during the following day's session, and it was joyfully received by the group as they danced and sang out along with Aretha. One of the women, JoAnn, formerly a math teacher from Detroit, had each of Aretha's four boys in her math class, and knew the singer well. Tears welled in her eyes as she lifted her arms to the sky in praise of the talented artist who gave us all so many years of beautiful, soulful music to enjoy.

With all the recent deaths from pancreatic cancer on my mind, I wanted to play another of Aretha's songs during that day's session, "Say a Little Prayer For me." But I didn't.

CHAPTER 41

Never Give In,
Never Give In,
Never, Never, Never!

—Winston Churchill

You may recognize this chapter title as another Churchill quote. When I'm feeling vulnerable, I try to keep the memory of this great man's courage in the face of tremendous odds uppermost in my thoughts. I'm not fighting a war, but I am fighting a battle, one that, so far, I'm winning. And, as the fearless leader had done, I "just keep buggering on," because the alternative is not an option in my favor.

I'm also remembering the advice of a dear friend, Nancy Green, who, sadly, passed away recently and is the friend who gave me that little dish with the words, "Look for Something Beautiful Each Day," inscribed on it. The dish sits on my kitchen table, propped against a colorful fruit bowl where I can see it every morning as a reminder to follow such wonderful words of wisdom.

Nancy, who was the director of our local theatre (CCAT), was instrumental in getting me the part in *Love Letters* and encouraged me to follow it through even though she knew I was barely recovered from the operation and chemotherapy. She believed in me when I was having self-doubts, and I am ever so grateful for her. That role led to another in Red Herring and to one I completed recently—an opportunity to participate in an annual theatrical musical event in Cambria called *The Follies*. Four months of dance, song, and scene rehearsals with the finest group of local actor/singers/dancers I could ever have imagined being part of. It was challenging but tremendous fun, and, if chosen, I am eager to be part of it again next year.

In the spirit of looking for something beautiful each day, I seek and find beauty in my garden where delightful little hummingbirds flutter from flower to flower, hovering every now and then to wish me a good morning. I find beauty in the books I choose to read—ones filled with heroic men and women throughout history, whether fact or fiction, such as *The Gentleman from Moscow, Adams, The Fountainhead*. I find beauty in the cherubic faces of young children, so innocent and joyful and full of an abundance of energy I wish I still had. I find beauty in the expertise of doctors, nurses, and researchers who tirelessly dedicate their lives to saving the lives of others. *Why are there no ticker-tape parades for them*, I wonder?

I find beauty in the hearts of friends and family who give their time and love and support so generously and who ask for nothing in return except that I do my best to survive. *They* are why I will never give in, never, never, never!

CHAPTER 42

"Cancer Is Cool...," Said No One, Anywhere, Ever!

I hope that if you or a loved one is coping with cancer (or any life-threatening disease), this book has brought you a little inspiration. If I have any words of wisdom to share that might help you in your fight to win this battle, they would be these:

🌱 **Grow!** Fact of nature: "All living things must grow or they will die." Every one of us will face death...eventually. But why help it along by standing still? Instead, learn something new to keep your mind active, to grow intellectually. Delve into a subject matter that is new to you. Read books in different genres. Audition for a play. Try a new recipe (Harold's pancakes follow). Take up a musical instrument. Learn to fly. Write a book?

❦ **Keep moving!** Especially outdoors. That's where most of life happens. Try pickle ball. Go skydiving or run a 10K. Take a trip. Start a micro-garden, fly a kite, or... as one pancreatic cancer survivor did, climb Mt. Kilimanjaro.

❦ **Laugh—maintain a sense of humor.** It really *is* the best medicine. (But chemo works, too)

❦ **Let others help you.** If you're stubbornly independent like I am, get over it! Friends and family want to help. Let them. Not because it will make you feel better (it will) but because it will make *them* feel better.

❦ **Indulge in your favorite things.** For me it included favorite books; Boni's burritos; my rose-patterned china; a green, silk pillow case, a burning fireplace; Dove bars; and a soft, *white* warming blanket.

❦ **Keep a diary about food, meds, and all reactions.** It will reduce the stress of having to remember what's needed on a daily basis and how you respond to each. It gives you an active role in monitoring your recovery.

❦ **Watch old movies,** especially musicals because they are so uplifting, and Westerns because the good guys always win...and you are one of the good guys.

❦ **Look your best.** If you're a gal, use makeup and wigs or scarves and hats. A guy, shave and dress in your favorite and most comfortable shirts, pants, shoes, etc. If you look better, you'll feel better.

❦ **Turmeric, turmeric, turmeric** (Ignore that it sounds like tumor, tumor, tumor). It's good for you. Check it out.

❦ **Stay on top of the news.** It's relevant. And, sometimes, good for a laugh.

❦ **Avoid conflicts of interest.** For instance, never read about cancer at the same time you're eating your favorite ice cream. (It's a downer, trust me!)

❦ **Take back your life!** Listen to "My Fight Song" by Rachel Platten at least five times every single day.

And, oh yes, be sure to *spend all your kisses*.

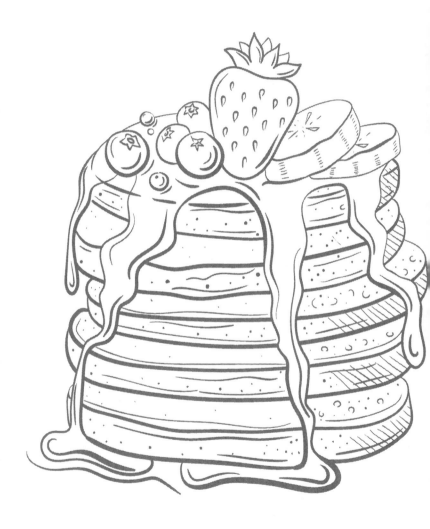

CHAPTER 43

Harold's Pancakes

In a large bowl, combine:
2 cups sour cream
2 cups buttermilk
2 eggs
In a separate bowl, sift together:
2 cups sifted flour
2 teaspoons baking soda
2 teaspoons baking powder
1 teaspoon salt

Add dry ingredients to wet ingredients until just combined.

Grill until bubbles appear on top, then flip the cakes.

Blueberries can be added into the batter for variation.

These are the lightest pancakes ever.

Enjoy!
Maryann
P.S. Using low-fat ingredients will not work as well.

Resources

The Pancreatic Cancer Action Network is the national organization creating hope in a comprehensive way through research, patient support, community outreach and advocacy for a cure. The organization is leading the way to increase survival for people diagnosed with this devastating disease through a bold initiative—The Vision of Progress: Double Pancreatic Survival by 2020. For more information, visit pancan. org or call 877-467-0875

The Hearst Cancer Resource Center (HCRC) at French Hospital is a one-of-a-kind resource in San Luis Obispo County for those living with cancer and their families, where all services are offered at no charge. The goal of the HCRC is to help those with cancer learn about the disease, recognize opportunities for improved health, build a personal support system, and gain a sense of extended family. The HCRC is dedicated to serving cancer patients and their families, ranging from those newly diagnosed with cancer, in treatment, in recovery, and beyond. For more information call 805-542-6234

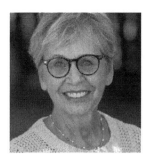

Maryann Grau was diagnosed with pancreatic cancer in 2016. The devastating effects of the disease were not unknown to her as both of her parents, and an uncle she had been helping to care for, had succumbed to one form or another of the disease. Additionally, both of her younger brothers are cancer survivors. The examples of courage, dignity, and humor demonstrated by beloved family members throughout their treatments were not lost on her, and she was determined to follow in their footsteps. Usually considered a death sentence—only 9% of pancreatic cancer patients survive more than five years—her diagnosis was no laughing matter. And yet, she credits her ability to write about her cancer experience from a humorous perspective as having had a major impact on her recovery. Maryann hopes that anyone facing difficult life challenges will read and draw inspiration from her book.

For more about the author, please interact with her at
maryanngrau.com

Made in the USA
Las Vegas, NV
01 November 2022